# LWW's
# STUDENT SUCCESS FOR
# HEALTH PROFESSIONALS
## *Made Incredibly Easy*

## Second Edition

**TOM LOCHHAAS**
Contributing Writer

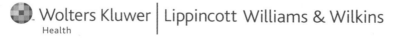
Wolters Kluwer | Lippincott Williams & Wilkins
Health

*Senior Acquisitions Editor:* David B. Troy
*Product Manager:* Renee Thomas
*Marketing Manager:* Allison Powell
*Design Coordinator:* Joan Wendt
*Artist:* Bot Roda
*Compositor:* Absolute Service, Inc./Maryland Composition

Second Edition

351 West Camden Street          Two Commerce Square
Baltimore, MD 21201             2001 Market Street
                                Philadelphia, PA 19103

*Printed in The People's Republic of China*

9 8 7 6 5 4 3 2 1

**Library of Congress Cataloging-in-Publication Data**

Lochhaas, Tom, author.
  LWW's student success for health professionals made incredibly easy. — Second Edition / Tom Lochhaas, Contributing Writer.
    p. ; cm.
  Student success for health professionals made incredibly easy
  Includes bibliographical references and index.
  ISBN 978-1-60913-784-7
  1. Health occupations students—Life skills guides. 2. Study skills. 3. Success. I. Olrech, Nancy. Student success for health professionals made incredibly easy. revision of (work) II. Title. III. Title: Student success for health professionals made incredibly easy.
  [DNLM: 1. Education, Professional—methods. 2. Health Personnel—education. 3. Achievement. 4. Vocational Guidance. W 18]
  R737.O47 2012
  610.71'1—dc22
                                                                      2010047410

### DISCLAIMER

CCS1210

# Preface

To reach their career goals, health professions students will travel through an obstacle course of classes, skills practice labs, and clinical rotations or externships. *Student Success for Health Professionals Made Incredibly Easy* is designed to help students through this process with practical study tips that will make them confident and successful students—as well as valuable members of the health professions team—by helping them understand the rules of the game and the skills and strategies they need to win it.

*Student Success for Health Professionals Made Incredibly Easy* uses the popular "Incredibly Easy" style to make learning enjoyable with a light hearted, humorous approach to presenting information. Hope, a health professions instructor, guides students through the book, offering helpful tips and insights. Along the way, she gets help from three health professions students: Amy, Anthony, and Leslie. Even when the tone is light, however, the concepts and tips are quite serious!

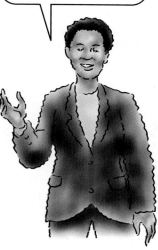

> Hi, my name is Hope, and I'm your guide to success as a health professions student.

## HOW THIS BOOK IS ORGANIZED

*Student Success for Health Professionals Made Incredibly Easy* is designed to be enjoyable to read, as well as highly informative. The book is divided into three parts:

- Part One presents basic principles for student success. Chapter 1 helps students get focused on academic success by setting their goals and anticipating obstacles. Chapter 2 focuses on managing one's time as a student—a skill that is increasingly important in today's hectic world. Chapter 3 covers basic issues related to health and well-being as a student, including how to prevent stress from hindering academic success. Chapter 4 then discusses the all-important world of interacting with others as a student, including getting to know instructors, networking with other students, and celebrating diversity.

- Part Two helps students sharpen their skills through several chapters focused on learning style and critical thinking (Chapter 5); improving listening, note-taking, and reading skills (Chapter 6); strengthening one's communication skills, including speaking and writing (Chapter 7);

> Congratulations on choosing the health professions for your career! I'm Amy.

mastering effective study skills (Chapter 8); and conquering tests (Chapter 7). All these chapters contain practical guidelines and tips for sharpening skills that will serve students well both in school and in their careers thereafter.

- Part Three chapters help students make the transition from school to their health career. Chapter 10 describes health professions while helping students identify how they will fit in best in their chosen career. Chapter 11 presents advice and tips for the clinical rotation or externship most health profession students will experience. Chapter 12 then explores how students can build on all their student success skills in the workplace—and the job application skills needed to get there.

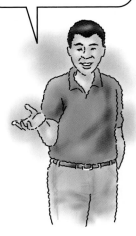

*Welcome, I'm Anthony. Glad you're joining the health professions team!*

## SPECIAL FEATURES

Each chapter of *Student Success for Health Professionals Made Incredibly Easy* includes special features designed to engage students with the topics and guide them in their study. Each can be identified by its unique icon:

**Winning Strategy**–kicks off each chapter with a list of objectives.

 **Playing for Real**–lets health professions students discuss how they put success tips into practice.

 **Tips from the Pros**–highlights important tips for student success.

 **The Finish Line**–wraps up each chapter with a summary of the key points.

 **Keeping Score**–presents review and critical thinking questions, along with chapter activities.

*Hi, I'm Leslie. You're off to a great start by using this book!*

In addition to these features, *Student Success for Health Professionals Made Incredibly Easy* includes both useful and practical illustrations and fun cartoons. The appendix contains answers to review and critical thinking questions.

# NEW IN THE SECOND EDITION

While retaining the popular *Made Incredibly Easy* look and student friendliness of the first edition, this second edition has been reshaped in several ways to make the book even more useful for students striving for success in their health care educational program:

- Much new content has been added in topic areas important for helping students master skills for success. Following are just a few examples of new materials in this edition:
  - more coverage of personal health, including avoiding substance abuse
  - financial management and budgeting—to ensure that students can afford to complete their program
  - involvement in campus activities
  - the importance of cultural diversity—and how to celebrate it
  - increased coverage of learning styles and tips for using one's personal style
  - fuller discussion of note taking, including the Cornell method
  - reading skills and finding one's way around a textbook and supplementary materials
  - guidelines for success in online courses
  - more information about health care professions, including personal and professional traits appropriate for different careers
  - increased discussion of the job application process and tips for success
- In addition, the second edition has undergone some reorganization to separate topics more clearly into groupings that can be taught in an individualized manner by different instructors. The change from 9 chapters in the first edition to the present 12 chapters is not a simple addition of three new topics but a reworking of the book's previous and new content in an organization that makes information easy to find, teach, and learn. The titles of chapters in the Table of Contents reveal this clear, practical approach.

## ADDITIONAL RESOURCES

In addition to the text, the following resources are available for students and instructors:

- An **Instructor's Resource Website** with test generator, PowerPoint slides, and Lesson Plans.
- A **Student's Resource Website** with printable note-taking guides for each chapter, printable calendar pages for effective time management, sample health professions cover letters and résumés, and other student activities.

All resources are available on the following companion website: http://thepoint.lww.com/StudentSuccess2e

# Reviewers

LWW would like to thank the following reviewers who added valuable insight for this second edition of *Student Success for Health Professionals Made Incredibly Easy.*

Jane Barley
Thompson Rivers University

Chris Haynes
Shelton State Community
College

Lea Hollenbeck
St. Louis College of Health
Careers

Tricia Leggett
Zane State College

Angela Satala
Triton College

Julie Skrabal
Bryan LGH College of Health
Sciences

Wendy L. Stone
Cortiva Institute—Boston

Patricia Sunderhaus
Brown Mackie College—
Cincinnati

Julia VanderMolen
Davenport University

Wayne Williams
South Texas College

# Contents

PART TWO
# SHARPENING YOUR SKILLS

## PART THREE
# ENTERING A HEALTH PROFESSION

# PRINCIPLES OF STUDENT SUCCESS

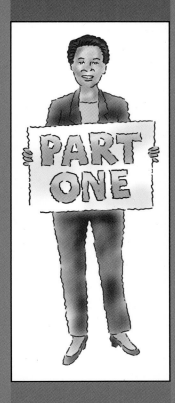

# Focusing on Success

*On completion of this chapter and the learning activities you will be able to:*

- List your reasons for wanting to continue your education

- Describe some obstacles that might limit your success as a student

- Understand why a positive attitude matters for success

- Practice staying motivated and focused on your studies

- Know the importance of goals

- Differentiate between short-term and long-term goals

- Set goals for yourself and make a plan of action to accomplish them

- Describe the three traits of good academic character

Way to go! By opening the pages of this book, you've taken a big first step toward your goal of continuing your education. In fact, you've already shown that you're motivated to succeed as a student!

The decision to continue your education may not have been an easy one to make. Maybe you haven't always had positive experiences with school. Or maybe you're worried about whether you'll have the time, energy, or money to stick with it. These concerns are normal— they're also shared by many of your classmates. By using the strategies explained in this chapter, you can gain confidence and sharpen your focus. Zeroing in on what you really want to get out of school will help you stay in the race and cross the finish line.

In this chapter, you'll take the first steps toward becoming a successful student. You'll think about why you're here—your dreams, the courage you've shown, the choices you've made, and the obstacles you've faced so far. You'll learn about what motivates you and about how to keep a positive attitude and stay motivated and focused. Most importantly, you'll learn how to set and achieve your goals while following other tips that will help you succeed in school. As a key part of success, you'll also learn the importance of maintaining a good academic character.

## WHY YOU'RE HERE

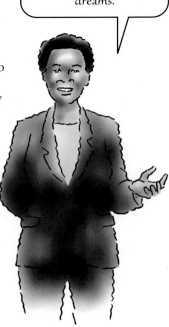

*Thinking about why you're here gives you reasons to go after your dreams.*

You may have just graduated from high school or perhaps you're returning to school after several years to start a new career. But, regardless of your age or experience, why is it important to think about your reasons for going to school? Because these reasons are where you'll find your motivation during those late night study sessions if you become tired and discouraged. Yes, even the best of students get tired and discouraged sometimes! And those are the times when it is most important to remember why you wanted to do this in the first place.

Taking a few minutes to be totally honest with yourself and really think about why you're here will give you a sense of purpose. A purpose that's personal and important to you will help you set goals for yourself. With real and reachable goals, you'll be more likely to succeed.

Student success means more than just passing your classes and earning your degree or program certificate. "Success," as it will be discussed throughout this book, also includes developing all the characteristics of a professional ready to practice in your chosen field. If that sounds like a lot, don't worry! This book will help you every step of the way.

### Dreams

What kinds of dreams have led you to this point? Maybe you're interested in finding a career you truly enjoy. Or maybe, you'd simply like to learn more about a subject that appeals to you. There are several reasons why people choose to continue their education. Do you have dreams of:

- improving your lifestyle? You may be the first in your family to attend college. If so, congratulations! The knowledge and skills you'll learn in school will give you more career choices.

- supporting your family? You may come from a single-parent home or you may be a single parent yourself. The ability to provide for your loved ones is an important dream to pursue.

- gaining self-respect? You may wish to continue your education to feel accomplished. Careers in health care provide both dignity and respect and are fulfilling work.

Whatever your dreams may be, they have brought you this far. Hold onto them and help yourself reach them by creating a plan for success!

## Courage

It takes courage to pursue your dreams. You've already shown courage just by being here! Stepping into the unknown is never easy, but you have taken the first step. Right now, school may seem full of unknowns. If so, know that you're not alone. Many students feel this way at first.

The best way to overcome a fear of the unknown is to become familiar with it. This book will answer questions you may have about school. You also will learn simple strategies to help you succeed as a student.

Remember that it takes courage to do something you've never done before. Taking this leap to continue your education will fully prepare you for other exciting things in your future.

## Choices

By choosing to continue your schooling, you are making your own path in life. It takes strength to make your own life choices and to work hard for what you want. Just as you've made a decision to continue your education, you can choose to have a positive attitude and be a successful student as well.

# OBSTACLES YOU MAY FACE

It becomes easier to overcome obstacles when you're able to recognize them. You may have overcome obstacles in getting this far. Let's explore this.

- What kinds of things have discouraged you in the past?
- How have people in your life helped or hurt your dream of going to school?
- What life experiences have influenced the way you see yourself?
- Do you foresee any obstacles in completing your education now?
- Do you feel confident you will be able to continue overcoming obstacles?
- Have you made a plan to overcome the obstacles you may face?

Recognizing the obstacles you've faced in the past will give you confidence to face future difficulties. You're probably stronger than you think! Although it may not be fun to face challenges, you can benefit from your experiences. If athletes never challenged themselves, there would be no championship games or world record holders. Overcoming obstacles helps you see your true potential.

Starting with this chapter, this book will help you develop student success skills to overcome both personal and academic obstacles that may arise between now and graduation.

# INGREDIENTS FOR SUCCESS: ATTITUDE AND MOTIVATION

Self-image affects your attitude and motivation. These two things are very important to your success as a student. If you feel good about yourself and have confidence, it is easier to develop a positive attitude and the motivation to learn.

## Liking Yourself as a Student

Of all of the factors that affect how well one does educationally, attitude is probably the single most important. A positive attitude leads to motivation and someone who is strongly motivated to succeed can overcome obstacles and succeed when others might give up or accept doing lower quality work. Your attitude toward education begins with your attitude toward yourself as a student. You may not have realized it yet, but you have become a new person. You're not just the same old person who happens now to be taking courses.

What do you think of this new person? Do you like him or her?

If you're feeling excited and enthusiastic, capable and confident in your new life, great! But if you are feeling any doubts, take comfort in knowing that you're not alone. A lot of new students worry, "I'm not a good enough student" or "I can't keep up with all this." Some may become fearful or apathetic.

An attitude that is less than positive, however, can hinder your motivation and ability to succeed. If you think you can't make it, that might become true. This is called a "self-fulfilling prophecy," and psychologists have shown it happens often. For example, if you do not do well on a particular test, you might start thinking you're not very good with that class. Once you feel that way, your studying will be less productive, your attitude will be less positive and enthusiastic, and you'll set lower expectations for yourself. All these factors, then may lead to your not doing well on the next test; also, you will have made your own prophecy come true. But, on the other hand, if you tell yourself that you just weren't fully prepared for that first test but will do very well on the next, then your attitude and enthusiasm will contribute to more productive studying and you'll very likely do quite well. In the same way, you'll have made your positive prophecy come true!

If you sometimes have negative thoughts about being a student, think about why that is. Are you just reacting to getting a low grade on some test? Are you just feeling this way because you see other students who look like they know what they're doing and you're feeling out of place?

Some students also fall into a "victim mentality"—blaming their circumstances or other people if they are not successful. This is a kind of negative attitude that sets one up for failure. After all, if it's someone else's fault that things are difficult, then you can't expect to do well. Watch out for this kind of psychological trap! Now that you're in school pursuing your education, you have the same opportunities as others and can succeed on your own abilities once you know how.

The main reason why some students find it hard to succeed in their studies is that they haven't fully developed the right skills for succeeding in their education. So cheer up! You're on the right track right now to learn everything you need to succeed. This book will help you learn these skills—everything from how to study effectively, how to do better on tests, even how to read your textbooks more effectively.

Just remember that it all begins with a good attitude about yourself as a student. Remember your purpose—why you enrolled in your school or program to begin with—and stay enthusiastic.

## Does Your Attitude Need a Boost?

Your attitude often determines your performance in school. It's reflected in how much interest you take in your studies or how meaningful your work is to you. If you have a positive attitude about school, you will be better able to:

- figure out your responsibilities in the learning process
- set learning goals for yourself
- study for your classes in a more effective way
- improve your grades and performance as a student

What attitude do you currently have about learning? Find out by looking at some positive and negative examples of feelings about school. (See *Attitude Check*.)

Motivation is related to attitude and just as important. It's what makes you want to accomplish a task. As a student, the right motivation can help you:

- get started on projects and assignments
- meet deadlines without last minute stress

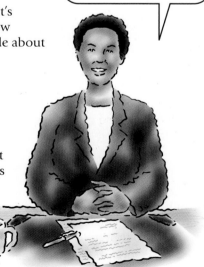

The secrets to becoming a successful student are having a positive attitude and staying motivated.

- move closer to your goals
- keep working on tasks until you succeed

Throughout this book, you'll learn how to motivate yourself to be a successful student, starting with the next section.

---

**Attitude Check**

Is your learning attitude positive or negative?

| *Positive* | *Negative* |
|---|---|
| • I'm good at studying. I focus well. | • It's hard for me to study. I get distracted easily. |
| • I enjoy learning new things no matter what the subject may be. | • I enjoy learning only about subjects that interest me. |
| • It's easy for me to learn new information. | • It's hard for me to process new information. |
| • If the instructor doesn't tell me what to study, I'll develop my own studying strategy. | • If the instructor doesn't tell me what to study, I'm often lost. |
| • I'm confident that I can learn and succeed. | • I'm doubtful about my ability to learn and succeed. |
| • I have a support system of family, friends, and coworkers—and I rely on them often! | • I don't like to ask people for help and I don't have a good support system. |
| • I exercise my mind, as well as my body, on a regular basis. | • I don't have time to exercise and I'd rather watch TV than read a book. |
| • I consider myself an optimist. | • I consider myself a pessimist. |

If you have more negative traits than positive, don't be discouraged! Recognizing a negative attitude is the first step toward changing it.

---

## ATTITUDE READJUSTMENT

If you find it difficult sometimes to maintain a positive attitude, there are many things you can do to help get back on track. Here are just a few that have proven to work:

- *Talk positively to yourself.* We all have conversations with ourselves. You might not have been successful on a test and start saying to yourself, "I'm just not smart enough" or "That teacher is so hard, no one could pass that test." The problem when we talk to ourselves this way is that we listen—and we start believing what we're hearing. Then our attitude becomes negative. Instead, have upbeat conversations with yourself. Say, "I've been paying attention in class and doing my homework and I just know I'm going to ace that test!"

- *Spend time with positive people.* If you notice that the people you're hanging out with tend to complain a lot and blame others for their problems, it's time for a change. Spend some time with other students who are happy with themselves as students. A positive attitude is contagious! It's also more fun to be with people who are upbeat and enjoying life.

- *Overcome resistance to change.* You're no doubt very busy in your new life and probably many things have changed for you. Sometimes we're slow to accept change and our attitude can become negative if we're always looking back. Consider instead your positive changes: the exciting and interesting people you're meeting, the education you're getting that will lead to a bright future, and the challenges and stimulation you're feeling every day. The first step in overcoming resistance to change may be simply to see yourself succeeding in your new life. Visualize yourself as a student taking control, enjoying classes, studying effectively, and getting good grades.

- *Overcome fears.* One of the most common fears students have is a fear of failure—of not making the grade. Life is not all roses and we all know we won't succeed at everything we try—and everyone has fears. The question is what one does about it. If you worry about not succeeding, turn that fear around and use it in a positive way. If you're afraid you may not do well on an upcoming exam, don't mope around. Instead, sit down and schedule your studying well ahead of time. Think of all the times you've been successful and tell yourself you'll do it again now. With that attitude adjustment, you'll more easily find you can!

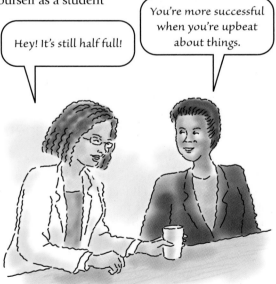

## Your Cheering Section

As a student beginning a new education, it's important to surround yourself with people who love and support you. A strong support system helps you maintain a winning attitude. And a winning attitude will put you ahead of the game in school!

To become a successful student, seek out support from people and resources such as:

- friends and family
- coworkers
- other students
- campus discussion groups
- instructors and tutors
- academic advisors
- student support services
- campus resources (libraries, computer labs, writing centers, etc.)

To maintain good relationships, be sure to discuss with your family and friends how things are changing while you're in school. Because of your new schedule, you may find that you need extra help with household chores or running errands. If you have young children, be sure to explain your schedule changes to them as well. Let your family and friends know that these demands on your time aren't permanent and that you're going to need their help while you're in school. Make these discussions positive and upbeat so that your family and friends feel good about how they're supporting your success as a student!

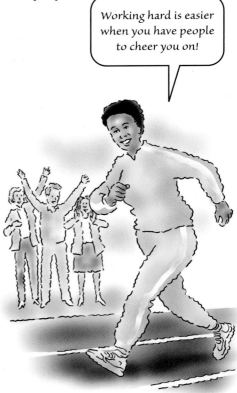

*Working hard is easier when you have people to cheer you on!*

## Uncertainty, Fear, Discouragement— Stop the Cycle!

If you feel uncertain or fearful about school, you won't perform as well and then you'll feel even more discouraged. This becomes a self-reinforcing cycle that can spiral further downward. By developing a positive attitude about learning, however, you can replace this with a cycle of self confidence, strong performance, and success. Here's how:

- Take responsibility for your education. Don't simply rely on others to teach you. If a class becomes difficult, ask for help! Your instructor, a tutor, or a classmate may be able to explain difficult concepts.

- Be an active learner. Ask questions about things that interest you. Look for ways to expand your education beyond time spent in the classroom.

• Decide what you want to learn from each course. Evaluate what courses you are enjoying most and, if you identify an area of difficulty, you may want to think about whether a particular degree or certificate plan is right for you. (In Chapter 10, you'll learn how to match your interests and abilities with the right health care career.)

Stress can be another cause of discouragement. When it seems like you have too much work to do and not enough time, stress can be overwhelming. Everyone experiences stress at one point or another. The good news is that there are many different ways of handling stress. Choose a method that works best for you. How well you manage stress will determine how much it affects your performance as a student. When stress is managed well overall, small amounts of stress actually help you stay focused and complete tasks. Don't let stress control you. Instead, take control of stress! (Chapter 3 provides some tips for managing stress.)

## You Can Do It!

To avoid discouragement, stay motivated. Use whatever motivates you to stay focused on succeeding in school. Your motivation may come from within yourself (intrinsic) or from outside benefits (extrinsic). Although intrinsic motivation generally can be more powerful and longer lasting (because *you* really want to accomplish the task), extrinsic motivation is also a powerful force. Take the Motivation Quiz to find out what motivates you to learn. (See *Motivation Quiz.*)

---

**Motivation Quiz**

1. I spend time studying for my courses because . . .
   a. I truly enjoy learning new information.
   b. I want to improve my grades and test scores.
2. I've chosen to go to school because . . .
   a. I want to excel at something.
   b. it will help me get a better job and a higher salary.
3. Going to school demonstrates to others that . . .
   a. I'm willing to take risks.
   b. I have an impressive résumé.
4. Learning new things . . .
   a. satisfies my curiosity.
   b. shows others I can get the job done.
5. I'm continuing my education because . . .
   a. I'm very interested in the subjects I'm studying.
   b. I'm looking forward to future promotions in my career.

If you answered mostly a's, then you're intrinsically motivated. If you answered mostly b's, then you're extrinsically motivated. If you answered a combination of a's and b's, then you're motivated in many different ways!

## THE FUN PART: CHOOSING YOUR MOTIVATORS

Once you know how you are motivated, you can choose your motivators. A motivator is a reward you promise yourself for completing a task. Choose one and then reward yourself for your hard work.

When choosing which motivators to use for school, think about the tasks you accomplish outside school. Where does your motivation come from? For example, if you volunteer at a homeless shelter once a month, what motivates you? Do you help out because it makes you feel good about yourself? Do you like to talk with the people you meet there? Do you enjoy helping others?

Understanding where your motivation comes from will help you choose effective motivators for school. If you are intrinsically motivated, it may be enough to know that you accomplished a task—and that you're moving steadily toward your long-term goal. If you are extrinsically motivated, you may want to promise yourself a more concrete reward. This can be as simple as having a nice snack after studying, enjoying a movie on the weekend, or buying a new laptop after successfully completing the academic term.

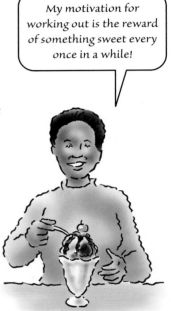

*My motivation for working out is the reward of something sweet every once in a while!*

## HOW TO STAY MOTIVATED

Okay, you've got a positive attitude. You're psyched! But you've got a lot of reading to do for classes to do tonight, a test tomorrow, and a paper due the next day. Maybe you're a little bored with one of your reading assignments. Maybe you'd rather play a computer game. Uh oh—now what? One of the interesting things about attitude is that it can change at almost any moment.

One of the characteristics of people who are successful is that they accept that interruptions will happen and plan ahead. Staying focused does not mean you become a boring person who does nothing but go to class and study all the time. You just need to make a plan.

Planning ahead is the single best way to stay focused and motivated. Don't wait until the night before an exam, for example. If you know you have a major exam in 5 days, start by reviewing the material and deciding how many hours of study are needed. Then schedule those hours spread over the next few days at times when you are most alert and least likely to be distracted. You also allow for time to see friends, see a movie, or surf the Web for a while to relax, rewarding yourself for your successful studying.

When the exam comes, you're relaxed, you know the material, you're in a good mood and confident, and you do well. You stayed focused and planned well and you had some fun along the way. Most important, you're maintaining a cycle of positive attitude and successful performance!

Planning is mostly a matter of managing your time well. We'll look at specific ways to do that in the next chapter. Here are some other tips for staying focused and motivated:

- If you're not feeling motivated, remind yourself why you're taking these classes. Remember the exciting career you're preparing for.

- Say it aloud—to yourself or a friend—with a positive attitude: "I'm going to study now for another hour before I take a break—and I'm getting an A on that test tomorrow!" It's amazing how saying something aloud helps you feel committed.

- Remember your successes, even small successes. As you begin a project or start studying for a test, think about your past success on a different project or test. Remember how good it feels to succeed.

- Focus on the here and now. For some people, looking ahead to goals, or to anything else, may lead to daydreaming that keeps them from focusing on what they need to do right now. Don't be too concerned about what you're doing tomorrow or next week or month.

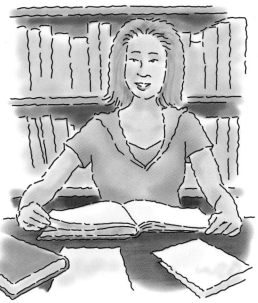

*It's easier to stay focused if you avoid distractions. Get away from your computer and phone—try the library!*

- If you just can't focus in on what you know you should be doing because the task seems too big and daunting (like sitting down to study for a final exam), break the task into smaller, manageable pieces. Don't start out thinking, "I need to study for the next 4 hours" (a plan that might feel depressing to many students), but think, "I'll spend the next 30 minutes going through my class notes from the last 3 weeks and figure out what topics I need to spend more time on." It's a lot easier to stay focused when you're sitting down for 30 minutes at a time.

- Never, ever try to multitask while studying! You may think that you can monitor email and send text messages while studying, but in reality, these other activities lower the quality of your studying and lower your motivation.

- Imitate successful people. Does a friend always seem better able to stick with studying or work until they get it done? What are they doing that you're not? *Visualize yourself* studying in the same way and getting that same high grade on the test or paper.
- Give yourself a reward when you complete a significant task—but only when you are done. Some people stay focused better when there's a reward waiting.
- Get the important things done first. When you're not feeling motivated, it's easy to decide you need to do your laundry instead of studying. Although cleanliness is important, this is a form of procrastinating and trying to fool yourself into feeling you're accomplishing something by doing laundry. Stay focused!

### Tips for Staying Motivated

- Keep your eye on your long-term goals to stay motivated with immediate tasks.
- Keep your priorities straight—but also save some time for fun.
- Keep the company of positive people; imitate successful people.
- Don't let past negative or less effective habits drag you down.
- Plan well ahead to avoid last minute pressures.
- Focus on your successes.
- Break large projects down into smaller tasks or stages.
- Reward yourself for completing significant tasks.
- Avoid multitasking.
- Network with other students; form a study group.

## BONUS BENEFITS

While motivating yourself to do well in school, you'll be accomplishing other things along the way. These long-term rewards may include:

- the ability to apply your study skills to other areas of your life
- a greater understanding of the course material
- confidence and an improved self-image
- better grades and test scores
- stronger performance in classes in the future
- better options in terms of salary and career

Motivating yourself as a student is a win–win situation. Not only will you be successful in school, but you'll be collecting short-term and long-term rewards along the way.

## The Balancing Act

You need to focus on your studies to do well in school. Worrying about money, your job, or other distractions can hurt your progress as a student. It can be difficult trying to balance all aspects of your life.

If you need to balance going to school with working full- or part-time, have patience with yourself. You can take courses at a pace that fits with your work schedule. You can learn time management strategies to create a manageable daily schedule that helps you maintain a good attitude and stay motivated. You'll learn about time management in the next chapter.

Distractions and other responsibilities also can be obstacles to developing a good attitude. Remember, you have to take care of yourself, too! Getting enough rest, eating healthy food, and exercising regularly will help you keep a good attitude. The better care you take of yourself, the better you'll be able to focus on reaching your goals.

Another way to avoid distractions is to set goals for yourself. By focusing on your goals, you will be less likely to become distracted.

*Start with smaller goals and move on to larger ones. If you wanted to become a mountain climber, you wouldn't start with Mount Everest!*

## SETTING GOALS

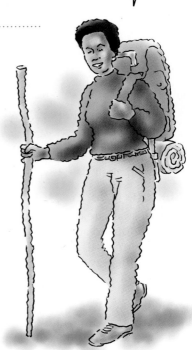

Setting goals for yourself is very important. It does, however, take a little practice. Some people are natural planners and can't help looking far ahead and, if you're like that, you may already feel comfortable setting goals and writing them down. But for those who like to dive right in and start "doing," goal-writing may feel frustrating and dull (at first!). But goal setting doesn't have to be complicated. Starting small will help you see how easy it is to write goals.

Begin by choosing goals that are simple and practical. By setting goals that are easily accomplished, you will pave the way for tackling larger goals in your future.

- An example of a good goal for right now might be to become familiar with your school's resources for helping students study. This goal is both simple and practical.

- An example of a bad goal would be promising to read your entire textbook before the first day of class. This is an unrealistic goal.

You should give yourself time by starting with smaller, more manageable goals. Once you have accomplished those, your goals can become more complex.

# Why Goals Are Important

Having goals helps you avoid distractions. Goals keep you from procrastinating, losing your concentration, and losing your motivation in school. In this way, goals are similar to the lanes on a racetrack. They help you stay on track as you run toward the finish line.

Goals come in many shapes and sizes. They can be small or large, easy or hard, immediate or future. Reaching your smaller goals will motivate you to keep reaching for your larger ones. Even completing a small task can give you a feeling of accomplishment. Overall, the more desirable a goal is, the more you'll want to reach it.

Goals should have three major characteristics. When setting goals for yourself, make sure they are:

- *Measurable.* All goals need a starting point and an ending point. Be specific. A goal such as "I want to complete all the assigned reading before each class this week" is more easily measured than "I want to be a good student."

- *Reachable.* Make sure your goals are realistic. Unrealistic goals can lead to discouragement. Remember, don't start with Mount Everest!

- *Desirable.* These are *your* goals. Make sure your goals reflect things you want for yourself. Also, make sure your goals are rewarding. Will reaching a particular goal give you a feeling of accomplishment?

# Long-Term Goals, Short-Term Goals, and Everything in Between

Goals can be divided into four main categories:

- long-term (5 to 10 years away)
- intermediate (3 to 5 years away)
- short-term (6 months to 2 years away)
- immediate (1 day, 1 week, or 1 month away)

### LONG-TERM GOALS

Long-term goals are often career or educational goals. These are things you hope to accomplish in the next 5 to 10 years. Consider your long-term goals as your finish line. Any other goals you accomplish along the way should help you make it to the end of the race.

### INTERMEDIATE GOALS

Intermediate goals are the next step below long-term goals. These goals are things you would like to accomplish in the next 3 to 5 years. If one of your long-term goals is to become a practicing medical assistant, your intermediate goals may include completing your education.

## SHORT-TERM GOALS

Short-term goals will help you reach your intermediate goals. Short-term goals are usually 6 months to 2 years in the future. If your intermediate goals include obtaining a degree or certificate, it may be helpful to have several short-term goals each semester or term, such as to excel in certain courses of particular importance to your program.

## IMMEDIATE GOALS

Immediate goals are things you plan to accomplish today, this week, or this month. These goals are small tasks that can usually be completed in an hour or less. Your immediate goals should help you reach a short-term goal. For example, suppose one of your short-term goals is to complete a lengthy research paper by the end of the semester. You can start by dividing the work into several smaller tasks that can be completed in an hour or less. These tasks could include choosing a topic, doing the research, making an outline, and writing a paragraph or two at a time. By completing these smaller tasks (your immediate goals), you will accomplish your short-term goal.

> At 3 to 5 years away, your intermediate goals may seem distant. Don't lose sight of them!

### Goal-Writing Exercise

Writing down your goals will help you stay committed and focused on reaching them. On the next page is a format for writing out your goals. Keep in mind that writing down your goals doesn't make them permanent. You'll be able to evaluate your progress and change your goals if necessary.

In addition, your long-term, intermediate, short-term, and immediate goals should all be linked together. For example, reading 20 pages of course material today (your immediate goal) leads to getting a good grade in the course (short-term goal), which contributes to earning your degree or certificate (intermediate goal), which in turn leads to the opportunity to become a practicing health care professional (long-term goal).

Long-Term Goal (to be accomplished in the next 5 to 10 years):

_____

_____

_____

_____

Intermediate Goals (to be accomplished in the next 3 to 5 years):

1. _____

2. _____

Short-Term Goals (to be accomplished in the next 6 months to 2 years):

1. _____

2. _____

3. _____

Immediate Goals (to be accomplished today, this week, or this month):

1. _____

2. _____

3. _____

Is each of your goals:

✓ Measurable?

✓ Reachable?

✓ Desirable?

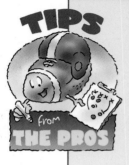

## Reaching Your Short-Term Goals

Short-term goals are things you would like to accomplish over the next 6 months to 2 years. Follow these steps to reach a short-term goal:

1. Write down your goal—the more specific you are, the better!
2. Set a reasonable deadline for your goal.
3. Think about possible obstacles to achieving your goal and how to avoid them.
4. Write down a step-by-step process to help you reach your goal—a plan of action.
5. Set reasonable deadlines for completing each step in the process.

## If at First You Don't Succeed, Revise and Try Again

Throughout the learning process, you may need to adjust your goals. Don't be afraid to make changes! Your goals are meant to serve *you*, not the other way around. They are not set in stone.

You may discover better ways of working toward your long-term goals. You may have to find creative ways of working around obstacles. Short-term goals can and should be changed to help you achieve success.

Along the way, you may decide to work toward an entirely different long-term goal. You may even be attending school without a clear long-term goal in mind. Once you decide to pursue a particular career path, you may reevaluate and possibly change your previous goals. If you find something you're passionate about, go for it! But don't be afraid to go back to the drawing board and change direction. Being excited about a long-term goal can be a great motivator.

> *If you miss a goal, don't punish yourself. Adjust your time line and keep going!*

### New Goals, New Future

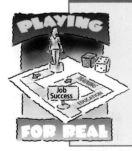

When I first started taking courses, my long-term goal was to become a radiologic technologist. Then I started working as a part-time administrative assistant in a dental office. I really liked getting to know the patients and seeing them every 6 months. The dental assistants in the office all seemed to enjoy their work. After one semester of school, I decided to change my long-term goal. My intermediate, short-term, and immediate goals all had to be adjusted. But I went back and revised my goals. Now I'm a certified dental assistant and I love my job!

### REWARD YOURSELF!

Rewards will keep you motivated as you work toward your goals. Rewards can be large or small, as long as they are appropriate for the tasks completed. For example, if you do well on an exam for which you've been studying for the past 2 weeks, it may be appropriate to reward yourself with a nice dinner out with friends. A large task deserves a large reward. However, it probably wouldn't be appropriate to reward yourself with dinner out every time you complete a 20-minute assignment! Maybe taking 5 minutes to listen to a favorite song would be more appropriate. In other words, smaller tasks deserve rewards as well, provided that the rewards are smaller.

## PEER PRESSURE AND PENALTIES

Another way to stay motivated is to tell a friend about your goals. Having another person to hold you accountable will put more pressure on you to keep working hard. In this respect, peer pressure can be healthy. Just be sure to tell someone who supports your goals. Encouragement from others can be an excellent motivator.

An unproductive form of motivation is punishing yourself for not completing tasks. Punishment often has the opposite effect of motivation. It can discourage you and affect your attitude in a negative way. If you miss a goal by failing to complete a task, try adjusting your time line instead. (See *If at First You Don't Succeed, Revise and Try Again*.) It's better to accomplish a goal a bit behind schedule than to become discouraged and give up on the goal altogether.

> Obstacles should make you adjust your game plan, not give up on your goals!

## Will This Be On the Test?

Grades help students measure their progress toward meeting their goals. However, a word to the wise: don't put too much emphasis on grades. Although that's easier said than done, in the long run, learning should be the true goal. Focusing on learning will help you grasp new information and then correctly apply it to situations in the future. After all, you won't be a very effective health professional if you don't learn the material in your courses!

Although grades should not be the entire focus of your learning experience, they can, of course, be great motivators. Achieving the grade you wanted on a big test that you studied hard for can help motivate you to study just as hard for the next one. Grades can also help you gauge your progress. You'll feel great when you see yourself doing better and better. On the other hand, if you're not getting the grades you want, you'll know you have to make some adjustments in your approach to your coursework.

To achieve your long-term goals, you may occasionally have to complete some school work that you don't enjoy very much. Maybe something that doesn't seem relevant. But stay positive even when you don't feel like completing these assignments. Although some tasks may seem dreary at times, you will always have the motivation if your main goal is to learn. Remember, if learning is itself a goal, you can more easily stay motivated to succeed.

## ACADEMIC CHARACTER

There's one more important topic for this first chapter, something you should be thinking about from your first day at school. What kind of person are you as a student? What kind of character will you have in your future career?

The character you have as a student is the character you'll have as a health care professional. You're facing the challenges of your new career today—learning new information, dealing with associates (the classmates of today are the coworkers of tomorrow), and taking responsibility for your work and your decisions.

Working in health care is different from working in most other careers. You are entrusted with patients' personal information on a daily basis. One day, you might listen to very private concerns, examine people's bodies, or handle their financial information. You must take these responsibilities seriously. People share information in a health care setting that they would never share anywhere else. You may learn things about patients that their own families don't know. The trust your patients put in you is critically important and sacred.

In school, you should develop the characteristics you'll need to become a trusted health care professional. Here are some main characteristics to work on:

*Your personal character matters when it comes to being a health care professional.*

- *Honesty.* Be someone your instructors, patients, and colleagues can trust.
- *Avoiding gossip.* Don't talk about other students, patients, or professional colleagues.
- *Accountability.* Be accountable for what you do at school and work all day, every day.
- *Responsibility.* Be someone who never tries to get out of doing work.

## Honesty

You should be familiar with academic honesty. It boils down to doing your own work: no plagiarism from books or articles, no copying a classmate's work, and no cheating on tests or assignments.

Honesty and ethical behavior have critical importance in health care. How would you feel if your doctor or nurse had passed a final by cheating? Or plagiarized their final paper? Or had a lab partner who did all the work for them? You would think that particular doctor or nurse was not qualified to answer your health questions or treat you. You would be right. Doing your own work is never more important than when you're learning to care for someone's health. You *must* know the material—you won't be able to fake it in a professional setting.

Make a concrete commitment to honesty.

- Do your own work.

- Avoid plagiarizing. Make sure you understand ideas well enough to put them in your own words.

- Own up to work you haven't done. If you're not prepared for a class or lab, admit it. Promise to make it up and that you won't let it happen again—and don't let it happen again!

Even though you are honest, you may find that some of your classmates are not. Take a stand here, too.

- Expect the members of your study group to do their own work.

- Don't let anyone copy your work. Sharing notes is not the same as letting someone copy an assignment you completed. Notes are raw material, not finished work that uses ideas and analysis.

- Don't let classmates force you to cover for them if they haven't done their work. You don't have to be confrontational, just firm.

Whenever you're in doubt about whether something you're doing is honest, think about it this way: would you want your doctor or nurse to do what you're thinking of doing? If the answer is no, don't do it. Period.

## Don't Gossip!

One of the biggest mistakes people working in a health care facility can make is gossiping about patient information. For example, suppose a coworker asks you a casual question about a patient. Even though it may seem like a harmless question, keep your lips sealed. Not only does sharing patient information violate the patient's privacy and the health care facilities policies, it can get you fired. (All health care workers must follow the privacy regulations of the Health Insurance Portability and Accountability Act [HIPAA], about which you'll learn more later.) You never know who is listening or where else that information might travel. Only share confidential information when it is required for providing care of the patient.

Even as a student, get in the habit of avoiding gossiping with other students. Even though it may seem harmless to chat about other students, gossiping can be habit forming, and talking about others now will make it more difficult to avoid later on in a professional environment. In addition to violating the privacy of others, gossip distracts people from focusing on the work at hand and can lead to conflict among health care staff.

Note that gossip and idle conversation about others extends also to your online presence in email and on websites like Facebook. Some students forget that even if they attempt to keep their personal information and image private when online, this information can be shared or become public in other ways. Make it your goal to present only a very professional image from this day forward!

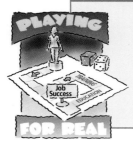

### No Bending of the Rules

I work at a local hospital on Tuesdays and Thursdays and the staff there know I'm a health care student. One day, a nurse's assistant was telling me about a patient of his. He likes to quiz me, so he gave me the patient's chart and asked me what I thought. It was tempting to show off what I've learned. But I gave the chart right back without looking at it. I reminded him of HIPAA regulations and told him I couldn't look at a patient's private information.

## Accountability

Being accountable means you have to be able to explain your actions. You are held to certain standards. An employee, for instance, is accountable to a supervisor. As a student, you are accountable to:

- your instructor
- your classmates
- yourself

You have to be able to explain to your instructor the quality of your work, your attendance, and your attitude. This means things like owning up to whether or not you studied and explaining why you turned in an assignment late.

How do classmates come into play? If you're working on a group project, you need to be able to tell the other group members about the work you've done toward the group goal—or why you didn't complete that work. You also need to be able to help everyone learn by participating in group discussions.

> Be a team player! Stay accountable to your classmates during group projects.

You're accountable to yourself in that you're working toward your own goals. If you're letting yourself down, you have to be able to admit it and then ask yourself why. You need to be honest in assessing your personal performance and behavior.

As a health care professional, you'll be accountable to:

- patients
- your supervisor
- your workplace

Helping patients is the reason why everyone at a clinic, doctor's office, or hospital is there. You are accountable to your patients.

When it comes to your supervisor, you'll have to answer questions about the work you've done. For example, a medical assistant might have to answer questions such as:

- Did you file all the paperwork?
- Did you check every vital sign?
- Did you label all specimens?
- Did you write down symptoms correctly and pass them on to the nurse or doctor?

And, more importantly, did you do all this correctly and on time?

Finally, you are accountable to your workplace—the health care facility where you work. Always work and act as though you might be called upon to explain your actions.

The way to make accountability easy is to toe the line. Do what you're supposed to do when you're supposed to do it. Be focused on your work when you're at work. If you form that habit now while in school, all the tips you learn about prioritizing and scheduling will come to your rescue after you graduate.

## Responsibility

Personal responsibility is key in school, work, and life. At school, you need to be responsible for managing your time, completing your work, and doing your best. As a health care professional, you will be responsible for all of those things and more—you'll be responsible for caring for patients, too.

Here are some things to keep in mind about your responsibilities at school and later in your career:

- You are responsible for your job—and only *your* job. It's great to help others when you can—you'll need the return favor some hectic day—but if others try to talk you into doing their work for them, politely refuse. Avoid adding tasks to your own. You may not be qualified to do them or they may be someone else's responsibility.

- You are responsible for your time—manage it well. Be able to account for it.

- You are responsible for your property—make sure you have the materials and supplies you need to do your job. Make sure everything is where you need it and clean up equipment and restock supplies after completing procedures.

- You are responsible for security and privacy. File sensitive patient information immediately and only share it with your supervisor.

- You are responsible for being educated and informed—keep brushing up on your job skills. Read professional journals, talk with colleagues, and ask questions. Ask to sit in on specific procedures if you need improvement. Review your old textbooks and make sure you know what you're doing. Participate in continuing education activities such as professional presentations.

- You are responsible for your actions—avoid the urge to blame someone else in a situation where your actions are being examined. Take responsibility for your mistakes. It's much better than trying to lie or shift the blame. Your instructors, colleagues, and supervisors will respect you for being honest.

All of these characteristics are being honed now while you're in school. Honesty, accountability, and responsibility are also the traits of a good student.

## CHAPTER SUMMARY

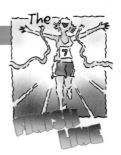

- One of the first steps toward student success is thinking about why you're interested in continuing your education. Your dreams are important in determining your goals.

- Learning to recognize and overcome obstacles will help you become a better student.

- A positive attitude and staying motivated are critical for achieving academic success. Work to develop a positive cycle of self-confidence and successful performance.

- Goals keep you from procrastinating, losing your concentration, or losing your motivation in school. Set goals for yourself so you can stay focused and organized.

- Short-term goals are usually set 6 months to 2 years in the future. These goals should help you reach your long-term goals, or career goals. Your long-term goals represent the things you'd like to accomplish in the next 5 to 10 years.

- When setting goals for yourself, make sure each goal is measurable, reachable, and desirable.

- Develop a good academic character as a student that will serve you well also in your future career. Be honest, accountable, and responsible.

## REVIEW QUESTIONS

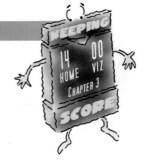

1. What are some common reasons why people choose to continue their education?
2. Write three to five sentences about how people in your life have helped or hurt your dream of going to school.
3. Name several groups of people or resources you could look to for support in your effort to be a successful student.
4. Explain the importance of a positive attitude for success in school.
5. List techniques you can use to stay motivated.
6. What three characteristics should each of your goals have?
7. Give three examples of problems that can occur in health care if professionals were not honest, accountable, and responsible on the job.

## CHAPTER ACTIVITIES

1. Get together with another student in one of your classes and talk about what you anticipate will be the most difficult assignment or project in that course. Discuss ways you work on it to ensure you are successful. Be sure to end on a positive, upbeat note showing your confidence in your ability to do it well.
2. Ask someone who has been out of school for years what they remember as the most discouraging experience they had as a student. Talk about how they might have prevented that negative experience with a more positive attitude, more motivated studying, and the use of motivational strategies discussed in this chapter.

## CHAPTER 2

# Getting Organized and Managing Your Time

*On completion of this chapter and the learning activities you will be able to:*

- Know why it's important to attend all classes

- Use all the class materials you receive

- Pay close attention to your syllabus

- Find and use campus resources that can help you succeed

- Develop effective time management strategies

- Get organized with a calendar, weekly planner, and to-do list

- Schedule and use your time effectively

- Recognize the symptoms of procrastination and take steps to keep on track

Attending classes is what school is all about, but being organized is also a large part of being successful in school. For example, your course documents will let you know ahead of time what each course will cover and exactly which assignments or activities your instructor considers most important. How you manage your time will also determine your success as a student. In this chapter, you'll learn how to use your course documents and campus resources to your advantage. You'll also learn how to organize your schedule and use your time efficiently. All these skills also help you stay focused on what really matters for success.

# ORGANIZING FOR CLASSES

Ultimately, attending your classes is most important for success. This starts with attending all classes, all the time, but also includes being organized with class materials and schedules.

## Being There

One of the most important steps in your student success game plan is to be there. This means attending all your classes, every day, beginning with the very first class. You have enrolled in your courses for a purpose. Missing a class here and there will make it harder to achieve your goals. Attending every class should be a top priority.

There are several reasons why attendance from the first day is essential. You will:

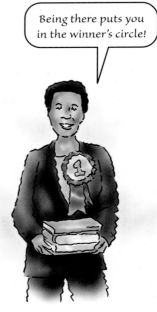

Being there puts you in the winner's circle!

- get to know your instructors and other students
- take notes if your instructors lecture on the first day of class
- find out about helpful campus resources
- receive important handouts so you'll know what to expect during the semester

Although some students think that nothing important happens in the first class and may be tempted to skip, that's a dangerous way to start the term! It's true that some instructors use that first day to introduce students to the course and then let class out a few minutes early. But many other instructors use the entire class time and start their lectures right away. They'll expect students to start taking notes on the first day. Missing the first class would put you behind in more ways than one.

Some students are also tempted to skip classes at the end of a term in order to spend extra time studying for final exams. But going to class should take priority. Instructors often provide their own review of the course and tell you which items or ideas will be covered on the final exam. If you schedule your study time well and stick with your daily and weekly schedules, you'll have plenty of time to study *and* go to class.

### WHY ATTENDANCE ALWAYS MATTERS

Class time is important because it gives you a chance to see the material you're studying through the eyes of an expert—your instructor. The instructor goes over key points, provides analysis, and brings ideas to life in real-world applications. In class, you learn what is most important for succeeding in the course and for entering your new career. Attending class needs to be one of your top priorities if your goal is to be a successful student!

Attending class means arriving on time (or even a few minutes early) and staying until your instructor has concluded the class and dismissed everyone. The first 5 minutes of class are just as important as the middle of the lecture. During this time, your instructor might make important announcements. The last 5 minutes of class are equally critical because your instructor might take this time to summarize important information or answer questions about an assignment. If you have an instructor who is occasionally late, don't use this as an excuse to skip the first few minutes of class. Instead, make use of the extra time by bringing other assignments or notes to review until your instructor arrives.

In school, showing up for practice means attending every class. If you practice enough, you'll be ready for game day!

Really, think twice before you miss a class. You joined the team—now you need to show up for practice. Each time you miss class, you fall behind. Even if you keep up with your reading and other assignments, when you skip a lecture or class discussion, you're missing out on an important part of the learning process. In class, the information from your assigned reading is analyzed and used as a building block for other, new information you won't get from a book.

Class time offers information you won't get anywhere else. It offers the instructor's own experiences and opinions on what you read in your textbook. During class, the instructor may share journal articles that discuss what you've read and take it further. Even if the instructor sticks to the textbook, you never know where in class discussion will take that information. You may hear a new idea during discussion that you never would have thought of on your own. Although some students think they can gain everything they need from borrowing another student's notes if they miss class, they will still miss the value of class discussion and interaction with the instructor. More real learning goes on during this time than can ever be captured in notes on the page.

Another important reason to make it a priority to attend every class: your instructor will notice if you skip a class or two. Instructors quickly memorize faces, even in large survey courses. They know when you're absent. And even if they don't pick up on your absence at first, if you go to office hours with a lot of basic questions, the instructor will inevitably take out the attendance log to see if you've been missing class. Even if attendance doesn't count in your course grade (it often does!), missing classes will affect your grade and make a poor impression on your instructors. It's a statement of how seriously you take your education and a measure of your desire to start a new career. If you take your classes seriously, your instructors will take you seriously.

**If You *Must* Miss a Class . . .**

- If you know you will miss a class, take steps in advance. Ask your instructor if he or she teaches another section of the course that you might attend instead. Ask about any handouts or announcements.

- Ask another student whose judgment you trust if you can copy their notes. Also ask if you can spend a few minutes with them after you've read their notes to go over things that may be unclear to you.

- You may not need to see your instructor after missing a lecture class and no instructor wants to give you 50 minutes of office time to repeat the lecture for you. But, if you are having difficulty after the next class because of something you missed, stop in and see your instructor and ask what you can do to get caught up.

- Remember the worst thing you can say to an instructor: "I missed class—did you talk about anything important?" This statement tells the instructor that you don't consider class time important—a major insult to the instructor!—and that you're not taking responsibility for your own learning.

## Using Class Materials

Attending every class is an excellent beginning, but being organized also means making effective use of course materials. Starting the first day of class, your instructors will give you various handouts and tell you about other materials you may need to access. These documents are critical for charting your path to success throughout the term.

### WHY ALL THE PAPER?

There's a reason instructors hand out so much paper at the beginning of the semester. They've spent the weeks before the first class planning every class session during the semester. They create a game plan of the material they're going to teach, the order in which it will be taught, and what you'll need to learn. Then they hand that game plan to you, in the form of course documents. Course documents help you get in the game quickly and easily.

Your course documents may include:

- a syllabus
- a class schedule
- a course materials list
- study guides or lecture outlines
- practice exercises
- assignment instructions

Course documents make life easier for you and your instructor. These documents help ensure that you're both headed in the same direction. This is very important for your game plan.

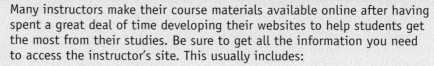

## Download This! Online Documents

Many instructors make their course materials available online after having spent a great deal of time developing their websites to help students get the most from their studies. Be sure to get all the information you need to access the instructor's site. This usually includes:

- the URL (web address)
- your user name
- your password

Once you have your password, keep it in a safe place. You never know when you'll need to go to the course website to review a course document. Also, if you happen to lose any of this material, you can print out a copy from the website.

## COURSE DOCUMENTS—GAME PLAN FOR YOUR CLASSES

For the most effective learning, you need to come to class prepared. You can find out exactly what's coming next by reading—and using—your course documents. In fact, reviewing course documents right away, at the beginning of the course, can sometimes help you decide whether or not to stay in a particular class. Look over the books and articles you'll be required to read. Consider how much time you'll have to spend in the lab. See how many exams you'll be taking and how much time you'll be expected to spend on homework. You may find that you've signed up for too many demanding classes during the same term. In that case, you might want to talk to your advisor about your course load and see if you should consider rescheduling one of your courses for another semester.

## SYLLABUS

The course syllabus includes key information about your class, just like a coach's playbook. Most instructors hand out a syllabus for their courses. The syllabus tells you almost everything you need to know about the course and what the instructor expects of you. A typical syllabus includes:

- the instructor's name and contact information
- the course name, catalog number, and credit hours
- when and where the class meets
- the goals your instructor has for you (what you will learn)
- the grading policy—how much tests, papers, daily participation, group work, and/or attendance contribute to your final grade

- information about whether the instructor will accept late assignments
- any special classroom rules

Most instructors will read through the syllabus in class on the first day and explain key points. Be prepared to highlight or mark these key points. This is an essential part of your first day, because you will learn about what each instructor considers most important. Some instructors place heavy emphasis on tests and papers, whereas others place a greater value on participation in class. As your instructor reviews the syllabus, you'll get an idea of what it will take to succeed in the course. Listen carefully to the instructor and be sure to ask questions about anything you don't understand. And, as with all handouts you receive, file your syllabus in a safe place right away.

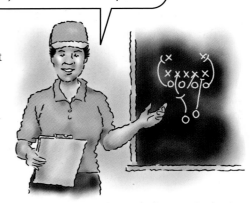

*Your instructor gives you a game plan in the form of course documents. Review these handouts so you know what to expect!*

## Staying Organized

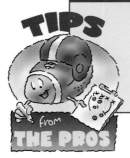

All that paper you receive from instructors is important! Look through it all carefully, organize it, and don't lose any of it. Set up a binder or folder for each of your classes. Place your syllabus at the front of the binder or folder because you'll need to refer to it often. Then continue to file all the papers the instructor hands out in class. You don't want to misplace any of your course documents or leave them behind in class!

### The Game Plan for Grades

Successful students have a game plan. They think through what they have to do to do well in their classes. They calculate what it's going to take to get the grade they want. This calculation often involves points or percentages. Unfortunately, many students find grades a source of confusion and frustration. They get their graded tests and assignments back, but aren't sure what the numbers really mean in terms of their overall grade.

This is another time when the course syllabus is very important: it will help you know how to figure out where you stand grade-wise at any time during the semester. But it may take some deciphering! For now, keep in mind that the syllabus has the information you need to figure your to-the-minute grade. In Chapter 9, we'll take a closer look at how to calculate grades.

## CLASS SCHEDULE

Usually, a class schedule is included with the syllabus and contains information about:

- what topics will be covered each day in class
- assignment due dates
- test and quiz dates

If the instructor has already organized the class schedule in calendar form, keep it in your binder for easy reference. If the class schedule is just a list of dates, get out your calendar (which you'll learn to make later in this chapter) and carefully write in the important dates. You might try using different colors, such as red for tests and blue for homework.

## COURSE MATERIALS LIST

The course materials list includes everything you'll need to participate in each class. This might include the following:

- *Textbooks.* If your school bookstore offers used textbooks for sale, this can save you a lot of money; just make sure you buy the right edition. Unless you must buy your books on campus, you may also find less expensive copies online—just be sure to order early enough that you have the book before class starts! Some textbooks come with CDs or an online component that your instructor may require you to use. Be sure if you buy a used textbook that it has the CD or online code with it. If you purchase your books before the first day of class, you will have a better idea of the material that will be covered in each course.
- Some schools offer used textbooks for sale at reduced prices. Because these books usually are sold on a first-come, first-served basis, it pays to purchase your books early.
- *Workbooks.* These may come with your textbook as a set or you may have to buy the workbook separately.
- *Photocopied readings.* Sometimes, an instructor makes handouts that he or she gives out in class. Other times, you'll need to retrieve handouts from the course website, the campus library, or the resource center. Be sure you have the course materials list with you so you get the correct handouts.
- *Uniforms, stethoscopes, etc.* The course materials list or your instructor will specify where to purchase these items. Ask if there are stores that offer special student discounts.

Sometimes an item on the list is recommended rather than required. Ask your instructor how important it is that you buy recommended items.

# GETTING ORGANIZED ON CAMPUS

Being organized and prepared doesn't end with attending class and organizing your course materials. Your success as a student is also enhanced by knowing about and using other resources on campus.

## Speaking the Language

Becoming familiar with your school and the resources it offers to students can be like learning a different language. Don't worry! There are people there to help you learn about things like course catalogs and financial aid. If you have questions but don't know who to ask, a good place to start is your school's information office. Look around at the more experienced students who seem like they have all the answers and remember that each of them had to start at the beginning, just like you! Trust that, in no time at all, you'll know your way around and be speaking the language like a pro.

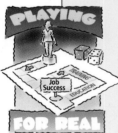

### Using Campus Resources

Hi, my name is André. I started taking classes a few months ago to become a physical therapy assistant. Going to school and working at a local restaurant keeps me pretty busy. I even thought about skipping the first day of class because I assumed it would be a waste of time. The instructors usually just talk about unimportant stuff and let everyone out early, right?

I ended up going anyway and I'm glad I did. My instructor talked about a lot of campus resources I didn't even know existed. He even gave us user names and passwords so we could access a free online tutoring system. It's been great! When I have to work an extra shift and don't have time to meet with my study group, I can log on and talk to a tutor. I never would've known about it if I hadn't gone to that first class. Being there on the first day has saved me a lot of time this semester!

## Course Catalogs, Credits, and Confusion

The college catalog or course catalog is one of the most important documents you'll use in school. It describes all of the classes offered in your program. It tells you about the requirements for your degree or certificate plan. And, it also helps you figure out when you will complete your education!

Your school may update the course catalog every year or every term. You should be able to get a printed copy or access the catalog online. Be sure to have an up-to-date version handy when planning your class schedule.

## TIPS FOR SCHEDULING SUCCESS

If you're attending a career or technical school, your course scheduling may be done for you. In other schools though, you may be responsible for registering for courses and organizing your own schedule. The way you organize your class schedule can affect your success as a student. A well-organized schedule ensures that you will be able to devote enough time to each course. There are a few tricks to organizing a schedule that works for you.

- Schedule your classes evenly throughout the week. You can accomplish this by scheduling classes every day. Overloading your schedule to have class every other day can lead to unnecessary stress. Distributing your classes evenly throughout the week will keep you from becoming burned out.

- Make allowances for tough courses. You can do this by scheduling tough courses when you are fresh. For example, schedule challenging classes in the mornings if you are a morning person. Another way to get through difficult courses is to balance your schedule for the term. Try to balance every difficult course with an easier one, if possible, so your schedule doesn't become overwhelming.

- Keep personal commitments in mind when scheduling classes. You may have to schedule your classes around work, family, and other obligations.

- Make informed decisions when choosing your instructors. Certain courses may be offered by several different instructors. When you have a choice, check with other students or your student government association for information on each instructor's teaching style.

## DON'T GET LOST—GET A MAP!

The first step toward becoming familiar with your campus is to locate a campus map. Maps may be found in the course catalog, on the school's website, or posted at different locations on campus. The school's information office can be helpful in answering questions about student parking and parking permits, if needed.

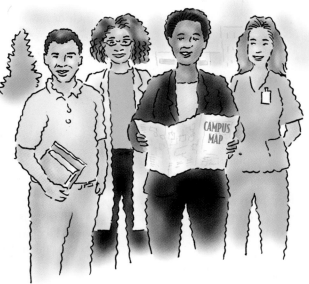

Knowing your way around campus can help you avoid unnecessary stress on the first day of class.

Each academic term, when you're taking new classes in perhaps new locations, plan to arrive a few minutes early the first week. Or, if possible, scout your classroom locations before the term starts so you know the route from the parking lot or bus stop and from class to class. It can be difficult getting used to a new routine and remembering where to go. Prevent unnecessary stress by giving yourself extra time to make it to your classes. It's better to be early and calm than harried, late, and out of breath!

## Campus Resources

There are a lot of resources available on most campuses that you may not yet have heard about. Most schools provide a variety of free services to any student who seeks them out, although it can take some hunting to find all of them. There are so many bulletin boards crammed with flyers advertising services and events that they can all merge into a senseless blur.

The fact that you also have to use your own initiative to find many free resources can be daunting. Who has the time and energy to track these things down? But, as usual, making the effort is worth it. Because so few students take the time to find all the resources available to them, there usually is an abundance of resources waiting for the person who does make the effort.

These resources and services can make a big difference in your student experience. Most are free for students or are already included in your tuition. Some of these services include:

- tutoring
- learning labs
- writing centers
- computer labs
- libraries
- fitness centers
- career placement services
- counseling

Need help revising a paper? Visit the writing center! Need access to a computer to do research or work on a report? Visit the computer lab! The people working in these labs and resource centers are often more than willing to help. Take advantage of their advice and expertise.

> Make the most of the resources your school has to offer.

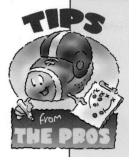

## Searching for Resources: The Starting Line

If you're having trouble finding out about the resources offered by your school, you probably just need to know where to look. Here are some tips to get you started on your search.

- Visit your school's information office and ask where you can find out about things like free seminars and learning labs.

- Ask your academic advisor to point you in the right direction. If you're struggling with a certain course, for example, your advisor may be able to suggest a possible tutor.

- Visit your school's website. You may find a "Student Services" section or a link to the Office of Special Services at your school and its list of offerings.

- Ask a librarian about resources available to students in the campus library. As a student, you may have access to special computer search engines, videos, and professional journal articles.

## THE CAMPUS LIBRARY

Although you probably know where the library is located, you may need to learn how to use the unique services available there. Your campus library has a wealth of resources: videos, books, articles, and other supplemental materials. Find out if there's a free orientation tour on how to use the library so you know how to find everything you need. Knowing how to use the reference area of a library is invaluable, but you may need to ask for help to use it effectively.

## LEARNING LABS

Libraries and learning labs are important campus resources. Most people know what a library is, but what's a learning lab? A learning lab is a place where students can go to meet with tutors or study groups, use campus computers, or use extra learning resources. These labs usually have very specialized learning material in them. For example, there may be life-size plastic anatomical models to help you learn anatomy. Some will have computers to aid you in learning how to use certain software programs. Knowledgeable people who can help you make the most of these specialized resources usually staff learning labs.

Find out if your school has a learning lab and, if so, find out where it's located before you need it. Remember, your goal is to be prepared. This saves you the stress of hunting for these resources later when you may be pressed for time.

## CAMPUS COUNSELING CENTER

The campus counseling center is also a good place to investigate. These centers often sponsor free seminars on studying, how to stay healthy, and how to manage stress. These can be great places to pick up information to share with your network.

> Find out whether your campus counseling center offers free seminars. There might be one that captures your interest!

## HUMAN RESOURCES

Don't think of resources only as offices and special rooms or buildings. The most valuable resources for heightening your learning are the people you see in your classrooms: your instructor and other students. Don't forget them!

In later chapters we'll talk about networking with students and forming study groups. Study groups can be among the most enjoyable—as well as most effective—ways to learn. You'll also be learning more about how to successfully interact with your instructors. But, from this point on, start thinking of your instructors as your most valuable resources.

### Help From Your Instructor

In addition to being available by phone or email, almost all instructors have regular office hours when they are available to meet with students one-on-one. You can go to your instructor's office and talk over anything you need help with. It's like having the instructor as your private tutor—for free! Find out when the office hours are (often on the syllabus) and write them in your schedule.

Check your class syllabus to see if you need to make an appointment for one-on-one time with your instructor. Also, keep in mind that office hours are for everyone in the class. Your instructor will have limited time to help you during office hours. If you feel like you need more help, such as weekly extended one-on-one tutoring, ask your instructor to recommend a personal tutor.

There are other options aside from meeting your instructor in his or her office. Some instructors offer help over the phone or by email. Some even set up online discussion boards. Remember not to assume that you can call your instructor at any time or that you can call as often as you want. Your instructor's time should be respected and shared equally with other members of the class. Be sure to call only during the appointed times.

If you send an email, you may not get an answer immediately. Most instructors will tell you what their response time is for email. Ask your instructor if he or she doesn't include this information in the syllabus.

## Special Services for Special Needs

Some students have special physical, mental, and learning needs. Special needs can include:

- physical disabilities
- mental disabilities
- learning disabilities

Most schools have resources to help meet these additional needs. For students with particular needs or disabilities, specially trained staff at the school can arrange for individual accommodations in the classroom. For example, students with hearing impairments may be able to apply for sign language interpreters to assist them. Students who have learning disabilities, such as dyslexia, can work with their academic counselors to find extra teaching and learning aids.

If you feel you need special assistance in school, you may need to seek out services yourself. Your school most likely has an office dedicated to helping students with special needs. Find that office to learn more about the resources available on your campus. If you aren't sure, set up a meeting with your advisor right away to find out what assistance is available for you. Although students are sometimes required to help pay for some of these resources, other times they are free.

# ORGANIZING YOUR TIME

A full-time student spends about 15 hours a week in the classroom and 2 hours of time preparing for each hour of class work. That's about 45 hours a week either spent in class or preparing for class. On top of these responsibilities, many students also devote time to their jobs, families, and other activities, along with time for exercise, socializing with friends, and all the other things you like to do. That's a full plate!

This is one of the things virtually all students agree on: there's not enough time for everything you want to do. But you can't "make" time, nor can you "save" it up for use later on. We only have so much time, so we have to learn to use it as well as possible. We need to be organized in our approach to time—this is called time management.

Time management is actually a set of skills. They are well worth learning because you can use them in your future career and throughout life. The better you manage your time, the less stress you'll feel, the more you'll get done, and the more time you'll feel like you have for doing those things you enjoy.

Here are some of the things involved in successful time management:

- knowing how much time you should spend studying
- knowing how to increase your studying time if needed
- knowing the times of day you are at your best and most focused
- using effective study strategies
- scheduling study activities in realistic segments
- using calendars to plan ahead and set priorities
- staying motivated to follow your plan and avoiding procrastination

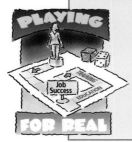

## Making Time Work for Me

My name is Angel. I'm 37 and I have two children. I work 30 hours a week at a bank and I go to school every day. My goal is to eventually become a certified nurse assistant. In a typical week, I spend 30 hours at the bank, 45 hours doing school-related work, and who knows how many uncounted, unaccounted-for hours making dinner, helping with homework, and doing laundry. I don't have a lot of wiggle room in my life. With so many responsibilities, I'm a typical student. Managing time efficiently is the key to my success.

## Where Does the Time Go?

We all have the same 24 hours a day, but some people just seem to have "more" time than others. How does that happen? Two different students might have identical amounts of homework in the same classes, work the same number of hours a week, and sleep and exercise in identical amounts, but one feels rushed and always behind in studying whereas the other feels calm and always has enough time to do a good job. What's the difference between them? Which type are you?

*I had no idea how much time I was spending just hanging out with friends!*

Chances are, these two students have different attitudes toward time. One may be more aware of time than the other—and therefore may be better able to manage it. Time management starts with being aware of where the time goes. Most people in fact often cannot account for how they spend all their time.

Accounting for and learning to manage time is so important for success as a student that it's worth spending some time learning to better understand time. Doing the following exercises and activities will give you a clearer idea where your own time goes. Step 1 is to see if you know how you actually spend your time day after day.

## Where Does Your Time Go?

See if you can account for a week of your time. For each of the categories listed, make your best estimate of how many hours you spend. (For categories that are about the same every day, just estimate for one day and multiply by 7 for that line.)

| Category of Activity | Number of Hours per Week |
| --- | --- |
| Sleeping | _____ |
| Eating and preparing food | _____ |
| Bathing, personal hygiene, etc. | _____ |
| Working, volunteer service, internship | _____ |
| Chores, cleaning, errands, shopping, etc. | _____ |
| Attending class | _____ |
| Studying, reading textbooks, researching (outside class) | _____ |
| Transportation to work and/or school | _____ |
| Organized activities: clubs, church services, etc. | _____ |
| Casual time with friends (include TV, video games, etc.) | _____ |
| Attending entertainments (movies, parties, etc.) | _____ |
| Time alone with TV, video games, surfing the Web, etc. | _____ |
| Exercise, sports activities | _____ |
| Reading for fun, other interests done alone | _____ |
| Talking on phone, email, Facebook, etc. | _____ |
| Other—specify: _____ | _____ |
| Other—specify: _____ | _____ |

Now get out your calculator and total up all your estimated hours. Is your number larger or smaller than 168, the number of actual hours in a week? If your estimate is higher, go back through your list and adjust your numbers to be more realistic. If your estimated hours total to less than 168, do not make any changes. Instead, ask yourself this question: *Where does the time go?* We'll analyze it to find out!

Step 2 in your time analysis is to actually track your time for a few days and see where you *really* spend your time. This may seem like a lot of work, but it really only takes a minute or two a day. The self-knowledge most people gain from this activity is well worth it and can pay off through all your time in school.

Make copies of the "Daily Time Log" (page 43). Carry it with you and every so often fill in what you have been doing (in 15-minute increments). Do this for several days and then add up the times for the different categories of activities in the earlier exercise on page 41. How does your actual time use compare with your earlier estimates? What have you learned about yourself?

Many students are surprised that they spend a lot more time than they thought just hanging out with friends—or surfing the Web, or playing around with Facebook, or any of the many other things people do. You can learn to use some of this time to your advantage! When you begin using a calendar or planner to schedule your study time the same way you plan ahead to attend class, you'll be on your way to efficient time management.

## Time Management Strategies That Work

Because you don't have all the time in the world, you want to use well the time that you do have for your studies. This approach promotes academic success while still providing enough time to enjoy life with friends, family, and other activities. Try these strategies:

- *Prepare to be successful.* While you are planning ahead for studying, think yourself into the right mood as well. Fight off any negative thoughts by focusing on the positive. "When I get these chapters read tonight, I'll be ahead in studying for the next test, and I'll also have plenty of time tomorrow to do X." *Visualize* yourself studying well!

- *Use your best time of day.* Different tasks require different mental skills. Maybe you can focus best on reading later in the day after you've burned off restless energy with some exercise. Maybe you can write a class paper more successfully earlier in the day when you still have a lot of energy. Some kinds of studying you may be able to start first thing in the morning as you wake, whereas others need your most alert moments at another time.

- *Break up large projects into small pieces.* Whether it's writing a paper for class, studying for a final exam, or reading a long assignment or full book, students often feel daunted at the beginning of a large project. That leads to a tendency to put it off. It's usually easier to get going if you break it up into stages that you schedule at separate times—and then begin with the first section that requires only an hour or two.

- *Do most important studying first.* When two or more separate things require your attention, do the more crucial one first. If something interrupts your work and you don't complete everything you planned to do, you'll suffer less if the most crucial work has been done.

- *If you have trouble getting started, do an easier task first.* Like large tasks, complex or difficult ones can be daunting. If you really

# Daily Time Log

## AM

| | |
|---|---|
| 5:00 | _____ |
| 5:15 | _____ |
| 5:30 | _____ |
| 5:45 | _____ |
| 6:00 | _____ |
| 6:15 | _____ |
| 6:30 | _____ |
| 6:45 | _____ |
| 7:00 | _____ |
| 7:15 | _____ |
| 7:30 | _____ |
| 7:45 | _____ |
| 8:00 | _____ |
| 8:15 | _____ |
| 8:30 | _____ |
| 8:45 | _____ |
| 9:00 | _____ |
| 9:15 | _____ |
| 9:30 | _____ |
| 9:45 | _____ |
| 10:00 | _____ |
| 10:15 | _____ |
| 10:30 | _____ |
| 10:45 | _____ |
| 11:00 | _____ |
| 11:15 | _____ |
| 11:30 | _____ |
| 11:45 | _____ |

## PM

| | |
|---|---|
| 5:00 | _____ |
| 5:15 | _____ |
| 5:30 | _____ |
| 5:45 | _____ |
| 6:00 | _____ |
| 6:15 | _____ |
| 6:30 | _____ |
| 6:45 | _____ |
| 7:00 | _____ |
| 7:15 | _____ |
| 7:30 | _____ |
| 7:45 | _____ |
| 8:00 | _____ |
| 8:15 | _____ |
| 8:30 | _____ |
| 8:45 | _____ |
| 9:00 | _____ |
| 9:15 | _____ |
| 9:30 | _____ |
| 9:45 | _____ |
| 10:00 | _____ |
| 10:15 | _____ |
| 10:30 | _____ |
| 10:45 | _____ |
| 11:00 | _____ |
| 11:15 | _____ |
| 11:30 | _____ |
| 11:45 | _____ |

## PM

| | |
|---|---|
| 12:00 | _____ |
| 12:15 | _____ |
| 12:30 | _____ |
| 12:45 | _____ |
| 1:00 | _____ |
| 1:15 | _____ |
| 1:30 | _____ |
| 1:45 | _____ |
| 2:00 | _____ |
| 2:15 | _____ |
| 2:30 | _____ |
| 2:45 | _____ |
| 3:00 | _____ |
| 3:15 | _____ |
| 3:30 | _____ |
| 3:45 | _____ |
| 4:00 | _____ |
| 4:15 | _____ |
| 4:30 | _____ |
| 4:45 | _____ |

## AM

| | |
|---|---|
| 12:00 | _____ |
| 12:15 | _____ |
| 12:30 | _____ |
| 12:45 | _____ |
| 1:00 | _____ |
| 1:15 | _____ |
| 1:30 | _____ |
| 1:45 | _____ |
| 2:00 | _____ |
| 2:15 | _____ |
| 2:30 | _____ |
| 2:45 | _____ |
| 3:00 | _____ |
| 3:15 | _____ |
| 3:30 | _____ |
| 3:45 | _____ |
| 4:00 | _____ |
| 4:15 | _____ |
| 4:30 | _____ |
| 4:45 | _____ |

can't get going, switch to an easier task you can accomplish quickly. That will give you momentum, and often, you feel more confident tackling the difficult task after being successful in the first one.

- *If you're really floundering, talk to someone.* A problem getting going on a project or large assignment may be the result of not really understanding what you should be doing. Talk with your instructor or another student in the class. Usually this will help you get back on track.

- *Take a break.* We all need breaks to help us concentrate without becoming fatigued and burned out. As a general rule, a short break every hour or so is effective in helping recharge your study energy. Get up and move around to get your blood flowing, clear your thoughts, and work off any stress that's building up.

- *Use unscheduled times to work ahead.* If you have a few minutes waiting for the bus, start a reading assignment now, or flip through the chapter to get a sense of what you'll be reading later. Either way, you'll be better prepared when you reach your scheduled reading time and will likely need less time. Use other down times during the day and you may be amazed how much studying you can get done in casual times.

- *Keep your momentum.* Remember to prevent distractions that will only slow you down. Save checking for messages, for example, until your scheduled break time.

- *Reward yourself.* Let's be honest; it's not easy to sit still for hours of studying or work on a special project. When you successfully complete the task, you should feel good about yourself and the reward of a (healthy) snack or a quick video game or social activity—whatever you enjoy doing—can help you feel even better about your successful use of time.

- *Just say no.* Tell others nearby when you're studying to reduce the chances of being interrupted. If an interruption happens, it helps to have your "no" prepared in advance: "No, I *really* have to be ready for this test" or "That's a great idea, but let's do it tomorrow—I *just can't* today."

- *Have a life.* Never schedule your day or week so full of work and study that you have no time at all for yourself, your family and friends, your larger life. Without a personal life, even the most dedicated student will suffer in a way that can negatively impact studies.

- *Use a calendar planner and daily to-do list.* We'll look at these time management tools in the next section.

# Calendars

People who manage their time well aren't just successful students—they're successful people. They take all areas of their busy lives into account and give each task the right amount of time and attention. The one tool successful people swear by is their personal calendar or schedule.

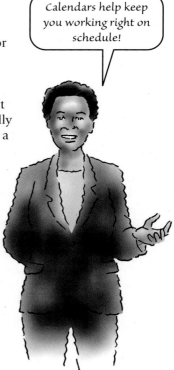

*Calendars help keep you working right on schedule!*

Using a calendar seems like a negative thing to some people. When they see those days fill up on the page, they feel trapped and overwhelmed. How will they get it all done? A calendar is powerful; it shows you exactly what you're doing each day and how busy you really are. But this is a good thing. Being able to see each week or month at a glance will show you days where you're trying to do too many things at once. A calendar shows you places where your time stretches too thin and emptier places where you can move some of those tasks.

Most importantly, a calendar helps you to be prepared. If something unexpected comes up, you can consult your calendar and immediately determine how that emergency is going to affect you. A calendar will keep you on track and help you remember important dates. Developing a personal schedule goes a long way toward fulfilling your time management goals.

As a student, you need to do both short-range and long-range planning. You'll need certain items to make this possible.

- a yearly calendar that you keep at home. This can be a paper calendar or an electronic version.

- a small weekly planner that you carry with you, adding new items as you hear about them. You can add the new information to your yearly calendar and check for any conflicts.

- a daily to-do list. You'll fill this list with items from your yearly calendar and/or your weekly planner.

You might choose to use an all-in-one organizer. Electronic organizers can store large amounts of information, yet they're small enough to carry with you wherever you go. Just be careful about keeping all your information in one place. If you lose it, you won't know your own schedule. It's always a good idea to have a backup, such as a yearly calendar at home that holds all your information. You can also find printable weekly and daily planner pages on the student website that comes with this book! See the inside front cover for access information.

## WHAT TO SCHEDULE ON YOUR CALENDAR—AND WHY

Don't think of your calendar or planner as only an academic planner. It is that and it has to include everything important in your life in order to work well, but you also have a life outside school. You need to include many important things to keep your schedule organized and avoid time conflicts. The calendar won't do its job for you if you mark next Tuesday's test but not your doctor's appointment scheduled for the same time. Put your whole life—work, school, home—on your calendar.

### Due Dates and Deadlines

Due dates and deadlines are usually stated in each course syllabus. These are very important! Turning in work on time helps you stay on schedule and keep up with the rest of the class. Although some instructors have special policies allowing for work to be turned in late, make a habit of turning things in when work is due.

### Tests and Quizzes

Test and quiz dates should also be marked on your calendar. Carve out blocks of time beginning several days before each test for studying. If you don't reserve time for studying, it could slip away from you. Prioritize your study time by scheduling it during a time of day when your mind is sharp.

Of course, you also have to prioritize attendance on test days. These are the "big game" days. If there is absolutely no way you can be in class on a test day (due to a family emergency, illness, or other circumstance beyond your control), let your instructor know as soon as possible and ask if the exam can be made up. Many instructors will not allow this, so if yours will, do whatever you can to make it up on the day provided.

### Projects and Group Work

When it comes to projects and group work, the scheduling isn't only up to you. As soon as you're assigned to a group, get together with your group members and block out times to work on the project. Start with the project due date and your instructor's recommendations of how much time you'll need to complete the work. Set aside times to work individually and times to get together.

It's tempting to leave this until later—why schedule time weeks in advance? But it's very hard to find one time when three or more people can get together. You and your classmates all have busy schedules. You'll have to prioritize your group work by getting out your calendars and determining a work/study schedule. That way, if someone tries to cancel, you can all remind that person that the date was agreed upon long ago and should be honored.

You'll also have more team spirit if you're working together according to a reasonable plan, rather than trying to cram in meetings with each other at the last minute or to assign work via email.

### Homework

Homework usually includes writing or reading assignments. Some students don't take homework seriously enough to include it in their calendar planner—they may think they'll "just get to it" eventually. But homework is actually a very important part of student success.

Written assignments show your instructor how well you understand the material. They show how much work you've finished and whether you know exactly what you're doing. Reading assignments don't give the instructor immediate feedback on your performance, but most instructors consider reading to be just as important as written work. You might see questions about reading assignments on quizzes or tests. Your instructor may base class discussions on the assigned readings. If your instructor relies on class discussions, be sure to complete the reading so you'll be prepared to participate!

When planning your weekly schedule, try to estimate how long it will take you to complete each homework assignment. This will be easier to do as you become more familiar with your instructors and your coursework. But at first, it's probably a good idea to add 30 minutes to your estimate. For example, if you think it should take you an hour to complete a homework assignment, schedule an hour and a half, just in case it takes longer. If you find it really does take you just an hour, you'll have 30 minutes to review, get started on something else, or just take a well deserved break!

Often, you will have homework based on an assigned reading or lab work. Try to get into the habit of doing the homework soon after the reading or lab work is done, when it's still fresh in your mind. The old saying, "Don't put off until tomorrow what you can do today," is never truer than in the context of homework.

## Field Trips

Field trips are invaluable opportunities to visit your future workplace. But they also can wreak havoc on your schedule. Do everything you can to make these trips. Your instructor probably will make clear to you how important it is to be there. Put field trip dates into your calendar so you can prepare for them in advance. You might need to:

- arrange childcare if you have young children
- take the necessary time off work
- ask your spouse or a friend to pitch in and help with any other responsibilities you may have on those days

Also, be aware that you may run late getting back from the field trip, so try to schedule some extra time for delays.

## Study Days

If your school schedules "study days" into each semester or term, plan to make use of these. Add these dates to your calendar well in advance. This will help you keep the days free as you schedule your other events and commitments. Try to avoid the urge to use your study days for any purpose other than studying!

### Other Responsibilities

Like most students, you probably have family, work, or other responsibilities outside of school. Sometimes, you might have to put off doing homework because of a more pressing obligation. This is understandable and, when this happens, it's okay to adjust your schedule. The key is to stay balanced. When you postpone working on a homework assignment because of another responsibility, be sure to make time in your schedule to complete the assignment before it's due.

### Time-out!

Whenever you can, try to create free time for yourself. You have to plan breaks if you want to avoid burnout—the fatigue, boredom, and stress that can make life miserable. A break can mean many things: switching from one task to another, getting together with classmates to discuss a group project, or moving from one subject to another.

You can also avoid burnout by keeping your daily schedule flexible. Be realistic when you're planning. If your calendar shows you have 3 days to complete an assignment, avoid trying to cram it all into 1 day. If you schedule commitments too tightly, you might not complete them on time (or at all), which can leave you feeling discouraged.

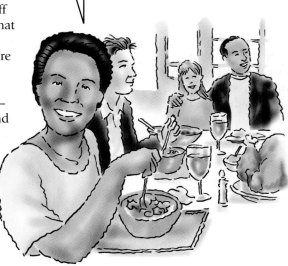

> Holidays are for relaxing and spending time with the people you care about. Try to complete your coursework before the holiday begins.

### Holidays

Holidays are times to relax and have fun. So make sure you do just that. It's tempting to put off coursework when you're busy, thinking, "I'll do that during vacation week." But vacation week often means your family is home, you're traveling, you're working so you can make some extra money, or you're getting together with friends. You won't want to spend that time trying to get work done—or failing to get it done. Block off holiday time and keep it free of any school obligations. You'll need that time to rest so you can come back refreshed and ready to get back to your schoolwork.

### Add/Drop Dates

You can avoid having to add or drop courses after the start of a semester by preparing properly before registration. Before you register for a particular course, gather as much information as you can. Meet with your academic advisor to determine the appropriateness of each course you plan to take. This way, you can avoid registering for courses you don't need. You'll also want to make sure you won't be taking several very demanding courses at the same time.

But even if you do everything right, you can occasionally run into snags after the semester begins. Maybe after attending your first few math classes, you find that it takes you a lot longer than you thought to complete the homework. It becomes clear that you won't have enough time this semester to devote to the class. For this type of situation, there is a solution—the drop/add period. During specific drop/add dates at the beginning of each semester or term, you can drop or add a course from your schedule without being penalized for it. Mark these dates on your calendar just in case this happens.

Keep in mind, however, that you need to be considerate of your fellow students. Often, there are students on waiting lists who need to take certain courses for their degree or certificate programs. Avoid using the drop/add period as a time to "test drive" courses. You may be taking a spot that someone else desperately needs! Instead, plan ahead before you register and avoid the stressful drop/add shuffle altogether.

## Last Day of Class

The last day of class is another important date to mark on your calendar. This date usually occurs several days before the start of exams. Although it's important to attend each class period, being there on the last day before exams is particularly important. Often, instructors review material that will appear on the exams and answer questions during this last class.

## Registration Dates for Next Semester

Approaching the end of one semester or term means it's time to prepare for the next! Mark registration dates on your calendar and give yourself enough time to prepare before registration begins. You might need to research certain courses or set up an appointment with your academic advisor to make sure you're on track for your degree or certificate plan. Remember, if you prepare properly before registration, you can avoid the drop/add hassle after the next semester or term begins!

It's also important to be prepared so you can register as early as possible. Required courses often fill up quickly. If you wait too long, you might not get into a course you need. Stay ahead of the game by going in on the first day of registration and getting it done.

Finally, don't forget about your finances. If you need to save money for the registration fee, you won't be caught unaware if you keep the date in mind.

## Managing Time by the Year

As mentioned earlier, you should keep a long-range yearly calendar as well as a weekly planner. You can use a traditional paper calendar or an online scheduling resource, such as the electronic calendars offered by free email providers. Use this calendar to record:

- class times
- midterm and final exam dates
- due dates for papers and other projects
- deadlines for completing each phase of lengthy projects
- test dates
- your instructors' office hours
- important extracurricular and recreational events
- deadlines for drop/add
- holidays, school vacations, and social commitments

### OFF TO A GOOD START

You'll probably notice right away that the beginning of each school term is a very busy and important time. During the first few weeks of a term, the instructor forms an opinion about what kind of student you are. Are you organized? Do you ask good questions? Do you know what you're supposed to do? Do you complete your work on time? Is your work done correctly? This kind of informal evaluation can help or hurt you. You'll want to be very organized from the start so you get a good reputation as a student.

Think of the beginning of each semester or term as a fresh start, or a new season. Just as athletes have the chance to prove themselves with the start of each new season, you can prove yourself a good student with each new semester. So start strong!

### A STRONG FINISH

A team that does well in the beginning of the season but loses steam before the championship game is soon forgotten. In school, you need to start *and* finish each semester with the same amount of hard work and dedication. The end of the term is important because you'll be running out of time to catch up if you've fallen behind in your work. Avoid letting your strong start from the beginning of the semester go to waste! Look at your calendar well ahead of time and try to clear less important events from the last few weeks of class so you can focus on a strong finish.

*Clear your schedule at the end of each semester so you'll have time to study hard and finish strong!*

## MANAGING TIME BY THE WEEK

Keeping a weekly planner helps you tackle the things listed on your long-term calendar, one week at a time. At the beginning of each week, you can plan for the tasks that are scheduled for that week. Here are some guidelines to follow as you create your weekly calendar.

- List regularly scheduled events and tasks first (such as class times, meal times, and the time you'll spend at work).

- Try to schedule time before each class for a brief review of your notes and to prepare for that day's lecture.

- When possible, allow yourself a few minutes after each class to review and organize your notes. Summarizing is a great (and quick!) way to review the material you just covered.

- Use your time efficiently by grouping similar activities together.

- Make it a habit to complete assignments before they're due. This way, you'll be able to turn in your work on time even if you come across snags in your schedule.

- Plan to study for 50 to 90 minutes at a stretch and be sure to allow yourself 15-minute breaks between study sessions.

- Base your study time on how many hours of class time you have each week. It's safe to estimate 2 hours of study time for every hour you spend in class.

- If possible, study at the same time every day. Choose a time when you're awake and alert.

- Use "gaps" in your schedule (such as time between classes) as study time. This way, you'll get more work done during the day and you'll have time to relax or do other things in the evenings.

- Schedule at least 1 hour per week to review how you will need to prepare for each class period.

- Be flexible by leaving some time unscheduled.

### Different Forms for Different Folks

A wide variety of planners and calendars are available for purchase or downloading from the Internet if you want to make your own. Is it better to have a separate page for every day—or a week spread over a two-page spread?

Sample planner page.

How should the time slots be broken down? This is all up to you. You'll soon find out what system works best for you.

It's usually best, however, to start out having *more* room on the page per day rather than less. If you don't have room enough to write down everything and to cross out items and add new ones when things change, then the planner can't do its job well and you may forget something important. The sample daily calendar page shown on p. 51 is just one student's preferred way of doing it, but it works well for this student. See what works best for you!

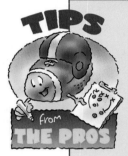

## Pregame Planning

It's best to create your weekly calendar on Sunday, before the week begins. Consider it your pregame planning session. Looking at the week ahead will help you spot any conflicts before they occur, so you can reschedule tasks as necessary. And being able to view the coming week at a glance will give you a chance to see how busy each day will be. Try to spread out your activities so each day is just as manageable as the next. You won't want to overload your schedule on Monday only to become burned out by Tuesday!

As you plan out your week, be realistic about the amount of time you estimate for each activity. In scheduling time for your commute to and from school, for instance, you should consider things such as the time of day and amount of traffic. If it takes longer to get to school in the mornings than it does to get home in the evenings, be sure to allow yourself enough time as you create your weekly schedule.

Other activities you should include in your weekly schedule are:

- homework assignments
- papers due
- upcoming quizzes and tests
- assigned readings

## Managing Time with a Daily To-Do List

Even though you have a weekly calendar with key information for each day, it's still a good idea to have a to-do list for the next day's activities. This gives you a game plan for the new day. Every night, check your weekly calendar and write down the next day's activities on an index card or small sheet of paper. If you use an electronic organizer, such as a personal data assistant (PDA), enter these activities into the next day's to-do list. Include things such as homework, study time, errands, and other tasks that are specific to that day—all the personal and academic tasks you need to accomplish that day. The tasks on your list should be specific and you should be able to accomplish them in the time you have. Include on your to-do list those little things not on your calendar that you still need to do, such as to buy a new cartridge for your printer, pay a bill before it becomes overdue, ask a friend to borrow a book—whatever you don't want to forget.

Keep in mind that you can switch certain items around as the day goes on if it will make your day more efficient. The point is to get everything done, regardless of the order in which you wrote the items down. Allowing yourself some flexibility will keep you from becoming stressed.

It's also important to reward yourself for accomplishing everything on your to-do list. Cross off each item after you've completed it. This will give you a visual record of your success. Giving yourself 5 minutes of free time for each large task you finish is another good way to reward yourself—and to make sure you don't overdo it.

Or try this: each day you complete everything on your to-do list, put a certain amount of money into a jar. At the end of the month, use the money to treat yourself. This works better than setting up punishments. Recognize achievement and use days you don't get everything done as opportunities to look at your schedule and to see what changes might make your days more efficient.

> I reward myself with some much-deserved free time after finishing everything on my to-do list!

## PRIORITIES

A big part of keeping a schedule involves managing priorities. Should you read an assigned chapter in your history textbook tonight or study for the anatomy test tomorrow? Both are important—both need to be done. But which is the priority right now? Setting priorities is important to your success as a student. You'll need to set priorities for tasks, class attendance, and homework.

As you'll learn in coming chapters, it's better to start early on big projects (studying for an exam, writing a paper, etc.) and spread out the work over time. Use your weekly calendar to schedule things well ahead of due dates to ensure you have plenty of less stressful time to work ahead. So even though you may have that anatomy test tomorrow,

> To do Today:
> • Study for anatomy test
> • Anatomy Test
> Read 20 pages for lab practical
> • Study group
> • Start research for lab assignment
> • Laundry

Sample planner page.

you ideally might have already studied enough for it and, instead of trying to "cram" tonight, you can do your history reading more leisurely and get to bed early!

It's all a matter of setting priorities and planning ahead.

## Making Progress

When you have several tasks with the same deadline, it's tempting to switch back and forth from one task to another. This feels like progress on all the tasks—they're all moving ahead. However, you're probably losing valuable time. When you switch from one task to another, you lose momentum. Your brain has to switch gears and begin thinking about a new project. Then, when you return to the first task, you often have to backtrack by finding out where you left off and what other steps need to be completed to finish the task.

### IN AN HOUR OR LESS

If you have an hour or less to work, your priority should be completing a single task as opposed to inching forward on several tasks. Here are a couple reasons why it's better to focus on completing one task when you're short on time.

- Completing an activity on your daily to-do list will give you a sense of satisfaction. Once you've crossed an item off your list, you'll have one less task to worry about completing!
- Completing a task moves you closer toward your goals. Think about it this way: Your instructors won't give you credit for simply working on a homework assignment, but they *will* give you credit if you complete the assignment correctly and on time.

### THOSE MARATHON PROJECTS

In the case of long-term projects, however, it's sometimes necessary to switch from one task to another. You can't expect to complete a 10-page research paper in one sitting! If you interrupt work on a long-term project to work on something else, write a few notes on the long-term project before you take a break from it. Your notes could include:

- the goal of the task
- a list of questions you need to answer
- the next step you need to complete

This way, when you come back to the long-term project, you'll be ready to get to work right away. Also, remember to keep all the materials you need for that project in one place so you don't have to spend time looking for them.

# PROCRASTINATION PITFALLS

Procrastination is the enemy of time management. Procrastination is so common that we tend to fall into its trap easily, thinking it's not so bad to put things off. But procrastination is just a fancy word for wasting time. And you know that wasting time harms your success as a student. It leads to missed opportunities, poor performance, low self-esteem, and heavy stress.

When you procrastinate, you spend your time worrying instead of working. The task you postponed starts to weigh heavily on your mind. You imagine how hard it will be and you start to dread it. But this doesn't have to be the case! There are several steps you can take to recognize procrastination and put a stop to it.

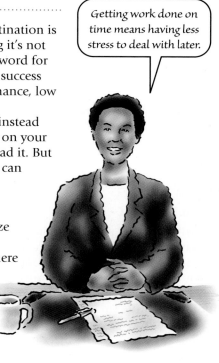

Getting work done on time means having less stress to deal with later.

## PRIORITIZE, PRIORITIZE, PRIORITIZE

One habit that leads to procrastination is failing to prioritize your tasks correctly. Putting low-priority (nonurgent) tasks ahead of high-priority (urgent) tasks is all too common. There are many familiar excuses for avoiding important work, such as:

- I'm not in the mood. I have to wait until I'm in the mood or I won't do well.

- I feel like taking a break to celebrate finishing one chapter. I'll read the second chapter after that.

- I'll do it tomorrow.

- I've got plenty of time—there's no rush.

- I don't know where to start.

- I like working under pressure.

- I need to do other things first or I won't be able to concentrate.

What's the thinking behind all these excuses? Often it's a lack of confidence. You might think the task is going to be too hard. You worry about being able to do it right. You fear it will take forever. You read every bit of material you can to "prepare" for the project—buying time before you have to begin. When you're worried about the outcome of a project, it's hard to find the motivation to get started.

Now's the time to shake off the lack of confidence that wastes your valuable time. First, remember who you are—a motivated, efficient student dedicated to your education and your future career. Then, remember why you're doing the project—to get the information and experience you'll need in your new career. Last, remember that nothing is as hard as it seems. You just have to start. The sooner you start, the sooner you'll be done!

Here are some ways to get started on that big project right away.

- Do a little bit at a time.
- Juggle your deadlines.
- Set realistic goals.
- Stay focused.
- Be confident about your decisions.
- Keep your goals in mind.

## A LITTLE AT A TIME

Try spending just 5 minutes on the project you've been dreading and putting off. Once you start, you'll probably find that you can keep working beyond 5 minutes.

## JUGGLING DEADLINES

Occasionally, the problem is having several deadlines in the same week. It's tempting to do the easier projects first, "leaving time" for the hardest one at the end of the week. But it would be wise to clear the most difficult project out of the way first. With the pressure off, you'll be able to relax a bit and work on the smaller projects.

If the projects are equally large, try parceling out the work. Set apart small tasks that can be done quickly for each project. Once you have those small tasks out of the way, you can focus all your energy on one project first, then the other. Completing several small tasks gives you confidence and gets you closer to being done.

## KEEP IT REAL

What if the problem is unrealistic goals? Some students don't start projects in time because they set standards that are too high (by accepting nothing less than 100% or vowing to do something better and faster than everyone else in the class). Then they're afraid they won't live up to those high standards. Or they won't stop working until they feel the project is perfect, which causes them to miss the deadline.

What is the solution? Weigh the consequences of handing in what you think is an imperfect project against the consequences of handing it in late or not at all. A passing grade for an imperfect assignment is better than a zero for not handing it in at all.

> When juggling deadlines, divide your work into smaller tasks to make it more manageable.

## BE CONFIDENT ABOUT YOUR DECISIONS

Uncertainty leads to indecisiveness, which usually ends in procrastination. For example, if you're not sure which topic to choose for a project, it becomes easier to put off starting the project. When this happens, remind yourself that you have to be decisive to become a successful student. Have confidence in yourself! The next time you're feeling lost and having a hard time choosing a topic, use these tips to help you get started.

- Brainstorm for ideas with other students.
- Ask your instructor for suggestions.
- Research several topics that might interest you.

## KEEP YOUR EYES ON THE PRIZE

Remember the long-term and short-term goals you wrote down in Chapter 1? By keeping these goals in mind, you'll have an easier time staying on track and avoiding procrastination. When you're thinking about your goals, an assignment becomes more than just another task that has to be gotten through. It becomes your ticket to reaching your short-term goal of passing the course. And passing the course moves you closer toward your long-term goal of eventually becoming a licensed professional.

By focusing on your goals, you can give yourself the motivation you need to complete assignments that you might otherwise put off. Review your goals whenever you feel the urge to procrastinate. Also, looking at your goals is a good way to get back on track if you notice that you're putting too much energy into one assignment at the expense of other projects and commitments. Your goals will help you stay balanced and moving forward to greater success.

## STAY FOCUSED

Where there's distraction, there's procrastination. Your mind will seek out distractions to avoid starting a project. You have to fight it. Get your game face on! Work on the project in a quiet area that is free from distractions. If you're in the kitchen, you might eat or do dishes as opposed to working. If you're in the living room, you might be distracted by the TV.

Another good way to avoid distractions is to make sure you have all the materials you need before sitting down to begin a project. It can be disruptive to your train of thought if you're constantly getting up to find another resource. Even small interruptions can cause you to lose momentum. Instead, gather your materials before you get started and then prepare to focus!

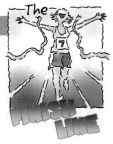

## CHAPTER SUMMARY

- Make it a habit to attend all your classes. You'll be a much better student.
- Use the course documents provided by your instructor to find out what to expect in each course you take.
- Investigate what campus resources are available to you, including your instructors and other students, to help you achieve success.
- Organize your time by creating yearly, weekly, and daily schedules.
- Schedule your time well for efficient and effective studying.
- Avoid procrastination by dividing large projects into several smaller tasks and setting realistic goals to focus on. Focus isn't something you have, it's something you do. In other words, you can *learn* to stay focused.

## REVIEW QUESTIONS

1. What can happen if you get in the habit of skipping classes?
2. How can your syllabus help you be successful in a course?
3. What items do you need to put into your yearly schedule?
4. Name several techniques for controlling your procrastination tendencies.

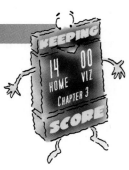

## CHAPTER ACTIVITIES

Planning Exercise: Work as a group to create a long-term calendar for a student taking the course for which you are now reading this text. Plan out the entire school term by referring to the syllabus or class schedule for information on:

- class times
- midterm and final exam dates
- due dates for papers and other projects
- deadlines for completing each phase of lengthy projects
- test dates
- the instructor's office hours
- deadlines for drop/add
- holidays and school vacations

## CHAPTER 3

# Maintaining Your Health and Well-Being

## WINNING STRATEGY

*On completion of this chapter and the learning activities you will be able to:*

- Understand how your health and well-being contribute to your success as a student

- Recognize the symptoms of stress and know how to manage it

- Stay healthy with exercise, good nutrition, and sufficient rest

- Know how to stay safe and avoid harmful substances

- Make and use a budget for financial well-being

When you're in school, you don't put life on hold. You still feel stress, or not, and you're healthy and happy—or not. If anything, health and well-being are even more important in school than at other times. You're likely to be stressed by a complicated life with many pressures. But you're also forming habits that you may carry forward into the rest of your life.

For all these reasons, it's critical to pay attention to your own health and well-being while a student. Stress can make you unhealthy, but good physical and mental health can reduce stress. Your overall well-being involves not only managing stress but also exercise, nutrition, and rest—the keys to good physical health—as well as maintaining personal safety and controlling your finances. Paying attention to all these dimensions of your life will contribute much to your success as a student.

# STRESSED?! WHO'S STRESSED?!?

The word *stress* usually carries a negative connotation. The dictionary defines it as "a physical, chemical, or emotional factor that causes bodily or mental tension and may be a factor in disease causation."

As you have probably experienced, stress can cause physical and emotional tension. It also has been linked to illness. These are all very negative effects. However, there are different types of stress and different reactions to stress. How you choose to manage stress can determine whether you have positive or negative reactions to it.

## I Stress, Eustress, Distress, We All Stress!

The two main types of stress are:

- *Eustress.* This type of stress causes positive reactions. Low levels of stress often motivate people to complete tasks, meet deadlines, and solve problems. You may encounter this type of stress every day. Eustress can be helpful. It can stimulate you to accomplish your day-to-day tasks.

- *Distress.* This type of stress causes negative reactions. High levels of stress often cause people to overreact. Distress can cause you to feel nervous and unfocused. It can hurt your ability to participate in and enjoy normal activities.

### SYMPTOMS OF STRESS

Identifying the symptoms of stress can help you manage it more easily. Recognizing stress at an early stage can help you keep short-term symptoms from becoming prolonged symptoms.

Some of these short-term symptoms of stress may seem familiar:

- You begin to take faster, shallow breaths.
- Your heart begins to beat faster.
- The muscles in your shoulders, forehead, and the back of your neck begin to tighten.
- Your hands and feet start to feel cold and clammy.
- You have a feeling of "butterflies" in your stomach.
- You feel physically ill, experiencing diarrhea, vomiting, or frequent urination.
- Your mouth becomes dry.
- Your hands and knees begin to shake or become unsteady.

*When managed correctly, eustress keeps me alert and focused. It helps me complete projects and meet deadlines.*

These short-term symptoms of stress are fairly similar for most people. They are also easily recognizable. Short-term symptoms stop occurring once you remove yourself from the stressful situation. For example, you may experience short-term symptoms of stress immediately before giving a speech in class. After your speech, however, your heart rate will return to normal and your palms will no longer feel sweaty.

Prolonged stress can have more damaging effects over time:

- Your immune system begins to break down as a result of lost white blood cells. You become sick more easily and more often.
- Free fatty acids are released into your bloodstream, which can clog arteries and eventually lead to a heart attack or stroke.
- Your risk for developing many different diseases increases.

The symptoms of stress are not always physical. Stress also can affect your mental and emotional well-being. Psychological symptoms of stress include:

- losing your ability to think clearly or remember things
- having difficulty solving problems
- experiencing anxiety or fear
- losing your ability to sleep through the night
- changing your eating habits—either eating significantly less or more than usual
- worrying
- becoming exhausted

With all these effects, it should be clear that stress can really get in the way of academic success. Fortunately, you can learn to take control of stress before it begins to affect you seriously.

## Taking Control of Stress

Just as there are different types of stress, there are different ways of dealing with stress. Several healthy ways of managing stress include:

- setting priorities
- simplifying your life
- learning to relax
- thinking positively
- gaining the support of others
- maintaining a healthy body

## SETTING PRIORITIES

Setting priorities means determining which commitments are necessary and which commitments or tasks aren't. Priorities help you manage your time wisely. By determining which activities are most important, you can avoid the stress that comes with trying to do everything. On a given day, your schedule may include attending class, studying, working, spending time with family or friends, and exercising or enjoying other hobbies. As you look at each task on your to-do list, ask yourself, "Is it absolutely necessary to get this task done today, or would it just be nice to get it done today?" Move the absolutely necessary tasks to the top of your list. After—and only after—those tasks have been accomplished, consider tackling the other items. If you're unable to complete all the tasks on your list, don't stress. Instead, feel good about everything you did manage to accomplish that day.

Prioritizing your activities allows you to feel satisfied with your accomplishments each day. If you find that some activities regularly fall toward the bottom of your list, you might need to cut those activities out of your schedule entirely. You may not have time for everything, but you can make time for the most important things.

## URGENCY OR EMERGENCY?

Another way to reduce stress is to adjust your schedule to fit your needs. If you have too many responsibilities that you aren't able to manage, try to give yourself more time. You may be surprised to see how many false deadlines you impose on yourself.

For example, if your coursework becomes overwhelming, consider taking fewer courses during the next term. It would be better to graduate several months later than to become overly stressed, break down, and wind up, unable to finish your degree or certification.

You can also avoid unnecessary stress by being able to tell the difference between an urgency and an emergency. When you feel stressed, divide your tasks into three separate groups:

- *Emergencies.* A task is an emergency if it absolutely has to be done immediately. For example, taking an injured pet to the veterinarian is an emergency.

- *Urgencies.* A task is urgent if it is important, but does not need to be dealt with immediately. For example, taking a pet in for its shots is urgent and should be done as soon as you have time.

- *Nonurgencies.* If a task is neither urgent nor an emergency, it is nonurgent. For example, whereas it is important to care for your pet, giving your healthy dog a bath is nonurgent.

If you have tasks that don't fit into any of the three groups, remove them from your list. They are not important and should be accomplished only if and when you have extra time.

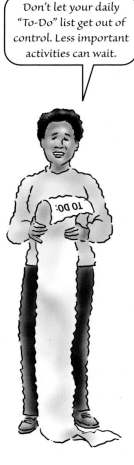

Don't let your daily "To-Do" list get out of control. Less important activities can wait.

## SIMPLIFY, SIMPLIFY, SIMPLIFY!

Because time is often short and most students have complex lives, simplifying your daily life can be another good strategy for avoiding stress. The following tips can help you simplify.

- Try to do all your errands in one place at one time. Going to several different locations may help you save money, but getting everything done at the same location saves you valuable time and energy.
- Don't watch TV every day.
- Let your voice mail take messages for you.
- Don't worry about sending greeting cards during the holidays.
- Stop attending functions you don't enjoy if they are not required.
- Avoid optional activities if they take up valuable time, such as chatting with your coworkers after work.
- Learn to say "no" when you have too much to do. Practice saying *no* to at least one request or invitation every week.
- Take time for relaxing when the job's done!

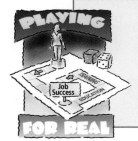

### Keep It Simple

As a massage therapy student with a part-time job, I find some weeks are more stressful than others. When school gets busy, I try to keep everything else as simple as possible. I do my grocery shopping and run errands before the week starts. After getting home in the evenings, instead of turning on the TV, I sit down, close my eyes, and relax. Even if it's just for a few minutes, it helps me feel less rushed. I also find that I get a lot more done on the nights I don't watch TV!

## RELAX INSIDE AND OUT

When you're stressed, your body reacts as if it's being attacked. Both your brain and the rest of your nervous system tense up. You can help back off from this "red alert" and reduce the stress you feel by learning to relax your body and your mind.

Try relaxation and stress management techniques such as massage, yoga, and meditation. Exercise is another relaxation technique. When you're sweating on a treadmill or pushing up a hill on your bike, exercise may not seem so relaxing. But after you finish your exercise session, you'll feel stronger, calmer, and more positive.

*Don't Forget to Breathe*

The next time you feel tense, try following this simple relaxation exercise.

1. Relax the muscles in your neck and shoulders.
2. Slowly lower your head forward.
3. Gently roll your head to the right and pause for 3 seconds.
4. Gently roll your head to the left and pause for 3 seconds.
5. Slowly roll your head down toward the center of your chest and pause for 3 seconds.
6. Switch sides and repeat, moving from left to right this time.

## MIND OVER MATTER

Stress can be caused or intensified by negative thoughts, such as worrying about school work or personal issues. To combat this stress, train your mind to focus on the positive. Try not to dwell on the stress you're facing. Acknowledge it and then move on to a solution. Focus on the goals you want to achieve and imagine how you will be successful. For example, you could start by acknowledging to yourself or a close friend that you're stressed about an upcoming test or the piles of paper-work waiting for you at work. Then, you could move on to a solution by making time to study thoroughly or by setting aside lower-priority tasks.

Remember that imagining worst-case scenarios can lead to anxiety and stress. Worrying is rarely productive. On the other hand, if you spend your time thinking about success, you will stay motivated to achieve it.

It's also important to spend time with people who can help reinforce your positive thinking. Family, friends, classmates, and others can help you stay positive and remind you that people care about you no matter what. Other positive coworkers can remind you that you're all in this together.

If you are unable to ignore your negative thoughts, try this meditation exercise:

1. Find a quiet place and sit or lie down comfortably with your eyes closed.
2. Begin to inhale slowly and exhale fully.
3. As you exhale, imagine that you are expelling the stress and negative thoughts from your body.
4. As you inhale, imagine that you are replacing the negative thoughts with encouraging, positive thoughts.
5. Slowly inhale and exhale until you feel the tension and stress fading away.

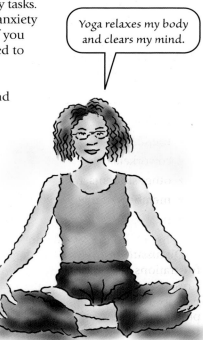

*Yoga relaxes my body and clears my mind.*

## Think Positively!

If you want to succeed, you should think like a person who expects success. Some ways to train your mind to think positively are:

- Say something positive every time you have a negative thought. You may want to repeat an inspiring quote or song every time your mind strays toward the negative. Little by little, you will overcome your anxiety.

- Get excited about upcoming projects and events. Imagine being successful in specific situations.

- Repeat positive mantras: "I *can* do this. I can *do* this."

- Be prepared. Have a "plan B" in case obstacles arise.

- Think of events that cause you to worry as learning experiences. You don't have to do everything perfectly as long as you learn something from your mistakes.

- Think of tests and exams as ways to demonstrate what you've learned. Don't get discouraged for not remembering everything. Completing an exam should make you feel proud and accomplished, not worried and inadequate.

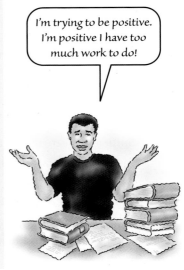

*I'm trying to be positive. I'm positive I have too much work to do!*

## NO MAN (OR WOMAN) IS AN ISLAND

The poet John Donne wrote, "No man is an island." There will be times when you'll need to depend on others for support. Having a network of supportive friends or family members will help you deal with stress. People in your network of support may include:

- family members
- friends
- coworkers
- other students and classmates
- members of religious groups
- people who share your interests in sports or hobbies

Discussing your problems or frustrations with others can help alleviate stress. People in your support system may be able to give advice or offer new perspectives. Surrounding yourself with people who care about you will keep you encouraged to reach your goals.

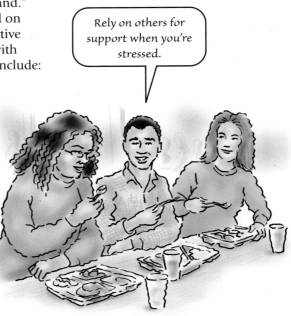

*Rely on others for support when you're stressed.*

# A HEALTHY BODY MEANS A HAPPIER YOU

As you are entering a health care career, you probably already know much about why good health is important. Taking good care of your body helps prevent many serious illnesses—and it also helps you handle stress more easily. Not least among the many reasons why good health is important is the fact that you'll be able to succeed in school more readily if you're healthy!

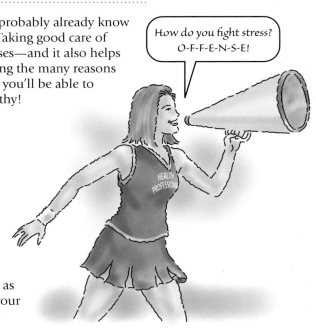

Four keys to good health are:

- Regular exercise
- A healthful diet
- Sufficient sleep and rest
- Avoidance of harmful substances

## Ready, Set, Exercise!

Exercising is an important way to keep your energy level up and help you feel good about yourself. Aerobic activities, such as running, swimming, or cycling, strengthen your heart and offer many other benefits as well. People who exercise aerobically:

- are less likely to get sick
- have more energy and mental alertness
- are less stressed and tense
- sleep better
- maintain an appropriate weight more easily
- improve their self-esteem

Choose an activity you truly enjoy. If you try to force yourself to do something you dislike, you won't be motivated to exercise on a regular basis. Another way to stay motivated is to exercise with a friend or in a group. Check around your campus for organized activities such as intramural sports, bicycle rides, a hiking club, etc.

If your daily schedule is busy, you may have to find time for regular exercise—add it to your weekly planner! Many working people, for example, exercise during their lunch break. Exercise may seem like a luxury, but it's a necessity for fighting stress and maintaining good health. If you take good care of your body, you'll be better able to keep up with your busy schedule.

For your body to receive the full benefits of exercise, you should work out at least three times a week for 20 to 30 minutes at a time.

For even greater improvement, work your way up to exercising four to six times per week. Just remember to give yourself at least 1 day of rest each week.

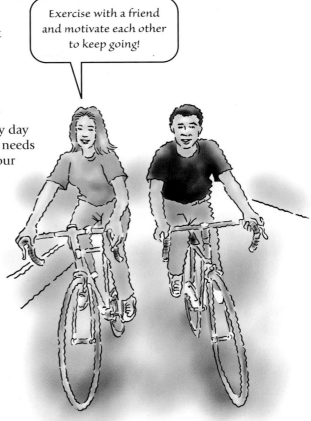

Exercise with a friend and motivate each other to keep going!

## Food = Fuel

Think of food as fuel. Eating breakfast every morning will prepare your body for the busy day ahead. You can give your body the energy it needs by eating healthy foods. This will prepare your body to deal with stress as well.

### FOOD FOR STRESS CONTROL

Vitamin B, vitamin C, and folic acid all help your body handle stress. These nutrients can be found in citrus fruits and leafy green vegetables, among other foods. And, the next time you find yourself reaching for something sweet to lift your mood, try eating foods that contain tryptophan instead, such as:

- milk
- eggs
- poultry
- legumes
- nuts
- cereal

Along with avoiding too much sugar, try to reduce your caffeine intake. Caffeine can cause tension and anxiety. Coffee, tea, and certain soft drinks contain caffeine and should be consumed in moderation.

### FOOD FOR THOUGHT

Your brain needs nutrition to function properly. Eating right can give you the strength you need and help you stay alert throughout the day.

Part of healthy eating also means having a balanced diet of vegetables, fruits, grains, and low-fat proteins. It's important to cut back on things like sugar, salt, saturated fat, and caffeine. Several cups of coffee each morning may seem like the best way to wake up and get moving, but caffeine can cause tension and anxiety. As a result, you may find it harder to deal with stress. If you're looking for an energy boost, it's best to rely on healthier options, such as eating nutritious foods, exercising regularly, and getting enough rest.

The key to keeping your body and mind in top working condition is to have a well-balanced diet. Electrolytes, such as potassium, calcium, and magnesium improve your physical and mental performance. Consider incorporating foods that contain these nutrients into your healthy eating plan.

Good sources of potassium include:

- fish, such as salmon, cod, flounder, and sardines
- vegetables, such as broccoli, peas, lima beans, tomatoes, and potatoes (with their skins)
- leafy green vegetables, such as spinach and parsley
- citrus fruits
- other fruits, such as bananas, apples, and dried apricots

Good sources of calcium include:

- milk
- yogurt
- cheese
- soybeans
- some vegetables, such as collard greens and spinach

Good sources of magnesium include:

- some fish, such as halibut
- dry roasted nuts, such as almonds, cashews, and peanuts
- soybeans
- spinach
- whole grains
- potatoes (with their skins)

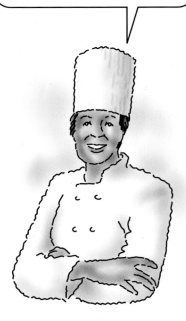

*Today's specials are a treat for the brain as well as the palate— a well-balanced diet with a side of electrolytes!*

## EATING FOR HEALTH

Eating right can be fairly simple. Just remember these basic guidelines.

- Make sure you include different types of food in your diet each day, such as vegetables, fruit, grains, and low-fat proteins.
- Check nutrition labels and look for foods low in saturated fat and cholesterol.
- Try to limit your intake of sugar, salt, and oils.
- Eat or drink caffeinated food or beverages in moderation.

- Drink plenty of water and avoid drinking too much alcohol.
- Balance the number of calories you eat each day with the amount of physical activity you do.

## Getting Enough Rest

Rest is also an important key to maintaining a healthy body. When you are well rested, you're able to complete tasks more efficiently. In contrast, feeling tired can increase the amount of stress you feel, which can wear your body down even more. Take cues from your body— when you feel tired, make sure you give yourself enough time to rest.

According to the National Institutes of Health, most adults need 8 hours of sleep each night. But, what if you're still unable to get a good night's rest even when you go to bed at a reasonable hour? Other things may be affecting your sleep.

- *Caffeine.* Do you often drink caffeinated beverages in the afternoons or evenings? Depending on how much caffeine you consume on a regular basis, it may be affecting your body's ability to rest at the end of the day. Caffeine is a stimulant that can stay in your system for 6, or even up to 12, hours. Your body may not be able to wind down properly in the evenings if caffeine is still affecting your system.

- *Nicotine.* Nicotine is a stimulant as well. If you're a heavy smoker, you may experience nicotine withdrawal during the night. Waking up multiple times can affect the quality of your sleep.

- *Alcohol.* Although having a glass or two of wine with dinner may make you feel drowsy, it can disturb your sleep later on. Alcohol can cause you to wake up during the night. As a result of drinking alcohol before going to sleep, you may wake up the next morning not feeling rested.

- *Food.* Eating foods that cause heartburn can affect your sleep. Not only does heartburn become worse after you lie down, it can interrupt your sleep during the night. Also, the amount of food you eat before falling asleep may affect the quality of your rest. Eating a large meal may make you uncomfortable and unable to sleep well. However, eating too little before bed also can make it hard to get a good night's rest.

On a positive note, a healthy diet and regular exercise can improve your ability to sleep. Making changes in those two areas may be all that's needed for you to start getting enough rest.

However, if you still have trouble sleeping, you may want to discuss it with your doctor. Getting good rest not only helps you manage stress, it's extremely important to your physical, emotional, and mental health as well.

## Sleep: How Much Is Enough?

When you're tired, you're more likely to feel helpless, incapable, and defeated. Nothing sabotages a positive attitude like fatigue. Make sure you get 8 hours of sleep each night. That may seem like a lot—another luxury—but it's necessary for your emotional, mental, and physical health. Sleep is key to good performance in school, at work, and in life in general. By taking courses, you've been asking yourself to do more each day, so it's a good idea to give your body the rest it needs. And getting enough rest will also help you do more in your job and make more of your career.

# Avoid Harmful Substances

"Substance" is the word health professionals use for many things people take into their bodies besides food. Although water and nutrients are needed by the body, these "substances" are not. When people talk about substances, they often mean drugs—but alcohol and nicotine are also drugs and considered substances the same as other drugs.

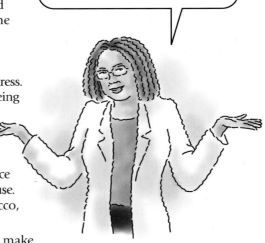

*Why would you want to put something in your body that will only slow you down and maybe lead to a real problem?*

Substances—any kind of drug—have effects on the body and mind. People use these substances for their effects. Some people use substances to try to alleviate stress. But many substances have negative effects, including being physically or psychologically addictive, and over time they actually increase one's stress. What is important with any substance is to be aware of its effects on your health and on your life as a student and to make smart choices. Use of any substance to the extent that it has negative effects is substance abuse.

The most commonly abused substances are tobacco, alcohol, and prescription and illegal drugs.

- If you don't use tobacco now, good!—but don't make the mistake some people make with "social smoking" with a friend, thinking there is plenty of time to quit later. Nicotine is one of the most addictive drugs in our society today—it will never be easy to quit. If you use tobacco now, start planning to quit by getting help. You might begin by downloading the booklet "Clearing the Air: Quit Smoking Today" at www.smokefree.gov.

- Alcohol is the most commonly used drug on most campuses. Drinking causes injuries to about 600,000 college students each year, resulting in 1,700 deaths. Almost 100,000 alcohol-related sexual assaults occur to college students. And about a fourth of all students report academic problems resulting from alcohol, resulting in lower grades. If you choose to drink at all, moderation is essential to avoid becoming a statistic yourself! Don't fall for the common myths about drinking not being all that dangerous. Learn more at www.collegedrinkingprevention .gov/CollegeStudents/alcoholMyths.

- People use prescription and illegal drugs for the same reasons people use alcohol. They say they enjoy getting high. They may say a drug helps them relax or unwind, have fun, enjoy the company of others, or escape the pressures of being a student. Like other substances, drugs have harmful effects on the body, affect one's judgment in ways that increase the risks for injury, and involve serious legal consequences if the user is caught. Why would any thinking student risk everything for a momentary high? If you have a problem using drugs, see a counselor at your campus health clinic for confidential help.

## HAVE A LIFE!

Don't let your busy life as a student prevent you from having a social life. People are social creatures and friendships and interactions with others help us all control stress—and just have fun! But sometimes students feel they are so busy with their studies and work that they should never take time out to enjoy the company of others.

School also offers the opportunity to meet many people you would likely not meet otherwise in life. Make the most of this opportunity! From social interactions you can gain a number of benefits:

- The emotional comfort of friendships with people who understand you and with whom you can talk about your problems, joys, hopes, fears—everything you feel—without worrying how they may react

- A growing understanding of diverse other people, how they think and what they feel, that will serve you well throughout your life and in your future career

- A heightened sense of your own identity, especially as you interact with others with different personalities and from different backgrounds

When you join study groups with other students, you get the best of both worlds: while enjoying the social interaction, you're also learning more and in more ways than when you study alone.

> Studying together is a great way to get some work done while still having some fun!

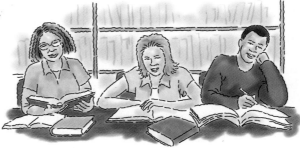

## STAYING SAFE

Your health and well-being as a student involves one more thing: personal safety and security. Although most campuses are very safe places, our world as a whole, sadly, is not always safe. Safety issues include preventing assault, date rape, and other violent crimes. By following a few common sense guidelines, you can stay safe both on and off campus:

- It's unwise to meet off-campus with people you don't know very well, especially after dark. Go to parties with friends—and stay with them to avoid becoming separated. Because date rape drugs are often added to drinks at parties, do not drink anything unless you know for certain it has not been tampered with.
- Don't give out your personal contact information (phone number, email address, etc.) until you have gotten to know a person well.
- Be careful if your date is drinking heavily or using drugs.
- Stay in public places where there are other people. Do not invite a date to your home before your relationship is well established.
- If you are sexually active, be sure to practice safe sex. Remember that most birth control methods do not protect against sexually transmitted diseases.

## FINANCIAL WELL-BEING

One of the most common reasons for students to drop out of school before completing their program is financial: taking on too much debt. This happens because some students simply spend too much and fail to keep a budget until it's too late, often taking on too much debt through credit cards and loans. True, school is expensive. But, by learning to budget and control your spending, you can avoid any more debt than is necessary to complete your education.

### Get a Job!

Most students these days work at least part-time. If you practice good time management (Chapter 2), you should have enough time for both work and school. Some students with greater financial responsibilities are able to work full-time while taking part-time classes.

Your school likely has a job office that will help you find a job if needed. The best jobs are those on or near campus, so you don't lose commute time, and those involving the school community rather than the general public. Working around other students and professors helps you feel connected to your school work and provides more satisfaction.

## Spending Less

Remember the exercise in Chapter 2 where you estimated how you spend your time—but when you actually monitored your time, you may have been surprised where much of it goes? The same is true of money: most people really don't know where it all goes. See how much you know about your own spending habits with the activity "Where Does the Money Go?"

---

### Where Does the Money Go?

Do your best to remember how much you have spent in the last 30 days in each of the following categories:

1. Coffee, soft drinks, bottled water                          $ _____
2. Fast food lunches, snacks, gum, candy, cookies, etc. $ _____
3. Social dining out with friends (lunch, dinner)        $ _____
4. Movies, music concerts, sports events, night life     $ _____
5. Cigarettes, smokeless tobacco                         $ _____
6. Beer, wine, liquor (stores, bars)                     $ _____
7. Lottery tickets                                        $ _____
8. Music, DVDs, other personal entertainment             $ _____
9. Ring tones, mobile phone applications                 $ _____
10. Fun techno-gadgets, video or computer games, etc.    $ _____
11. Gifts                                                 $ _____
12. Hobbies                                               $ _____
13. Newspapers, magazines                                $ _____
14. Travel, day trips                                     $ _____
15. Bank account fees, ATM withdrawal fees               $ _____
16. Credit card finance charges                          $ _____

Now, add it all up: _____

Be honest with yourself: is this *really* all you spent on these items? Most of us tend to forget small, daily kinds of purchases or underestimate how much we spend on them. Notice that this list does not include essential spending for things like room and board or an apartment and groceries, utilities, tuition and books, and so on. The greatest potential for cutting back on spending is to look as the optional things you spend your money on.

Because most students can't simply work more hours to provide a greater income, the better solution to avoiding debt is to learn to spend less. Follow these tips:

- Be aware of what you're spending. Write down everything you spend for a month to discover your habits.

- Use cash instead of a credit card for most purchases—you'll pay more attention.

- Look for alternatives. Buying bottled water, for example, can costs hundreds of dollars a year! Carry your own refillable water bottle and save the money.

- Plan ahead to avoid impulse spending. If you have a healthy snack in your backpack, it's easier to avoid the vending machines when you're hungry on the way to class.

- Shop around, compare prices online, buy in bulk. Buy generic products instead of name brands. Shop at thrift stores and yard sales.

- Stop to think a minute before spending. Often this is all it takes to avoid budget-busting purchases. With larger purchases, postpone buying for a couple days (you may find you don't "need" it after all).

- Make and take along your own lunches instead of eating out on campus.

- Read newspapers and magazines online or in the library.

- Cancel cable TV and watch programs online for free.

- Use free campus and local Wi-Fi spots and cancel your home high-speed connection.

- Cancel your health club membership and use a free facility on campus or in the community.

- Avoid ATM fees by finding a machine on your card's network (or change banks); avoid checking account monthly fees by finding a bank with free checking.

- Get cash from an ATM only in small amounts so you never feel "rich."

- Look for free fun instead of movies and concerts—most schools have frequent free events.

- If you pay your own utility bills, make it a habit to conserve: don't leave lights burning or your computer on all night.

- Use your study skills to avoid any risk of failing a class—paying to retake a course is one of the quickest ways to get in financial trouble!

# Managing a Budget

Most people don't use a budget to help manage their money—and most people in our society admit to frequent financial troubles. Could those two facts be related?

How can you know if you can afford to buy a new laptop or cell phone right now? Can you afford to eat out tonight or should you go home and cook dinner? Should you take that weekend trip? Will you be tempted to spend the money because it's there in your checking account? Or because your credit card hasn't hit its limit yet? But then, what about those textbooks you need to buy, or those groceries, or the utility bill that arrives tomorrow—will you have money for those things too?

Unless you keep a budget, you really can't know for sure. That seems so simple—but then again, *not* keeping a budget is why so many people have so many money problems. Using a budget is just like using a calendar to schedule your time: it keeps you on track. Managing a budget involves three steps:

1. Calculating all your monthly sources of income.
2. Calculating and analyzing all your monthly expenditures.
3. Making adjustments in your budget (and lifestyle, if needed) to ensure the money isn't going out faster than it's coming in.

This may seem time-consuming the first time you create and use a budget, but this is time very well spent—literally! Soon it becomes an automatic, easy process.

## STEP 1: CALCULATE YOUR INCOME

Use Table 3.1 to account for all funds available to you on a monthly basis.

| Table 3.1   **Monthly Income and Funds** | |
| --- | --- |
| **Source of Income/Funds** | **Amount in Dollars** |
| Job income/salary (take-home amount) | _____ |
| Funds from parents/family/others | _____ |
| Monthly draw from savings | _____ |
| Monthly draw from financial aid | _____ |
| Monthly draw from student/other loans | _____ |
| Other income source: _____ | _____ |
| Other income source: _____ | _____ |
| Other income source: _____ | _____ |
| **Total Monthly Incoming** | _____ |

## STEP 2: TRACK YOUR EXPENSES

Tracking expenditures is more difficult than tracking income. Some fixed expenses (tuition, rent, etc.) you should already know, but until you've actually added up everything you spend money on for a typical month, it's hard to estimate how much you're really spending on cups of coffee or snacks between class, groceries, entertainment, etc. You can start with the numbers you estimated earlier in "Where Does the Money Go?" Put these into the spaces in Table 3.2.

Note that there are *lots* of spending categories in Table 3.2. This is important—because, if you find you need to cut back your spending to stay on budget, you need to know *specifically* where you can make the cuts.

## STEP 3: BALANCE YOUR BUDGET

Now compare your total monthly incoming with your total monthly outgoing. How balanced does your budget look at this point? Remember that you probably had to estimate several of your expenditures. You can't know for sure until you actually track your expenses for at least a month and have real numbers to work with.

What if your expense total is significantly higher than your income total? First, you need to make your budget work on paper. Go back through your expenditure list and see where you can cut. Students shouldn't try to live like working professionals. There are many dozens of ways to spend less so that you can live within your budget.

It's normal to have to make adjustments at first. Just make sure to keep the overall budget balanced as you make adjustments. For example, if you discover that you have to increase what you spend for textbooks, you may choose to spend less on eating out—and subtract the amount from that category that you add to the textbook category. Get in the habit of thinking this way instead of reaching for a credit card when you don't have enough in your budget for something you want or need. That's your long-term plan for controlling your financial life.

If you want to get fancy and *really* take control, you can use a computer spreadsheet or financial program to track all your expenditures and manage your budget.

*Now I've saved enough for a new lab coat without having to go without eating for a week!*

## Table 3.2 Monthly Expenditures

| Expenditures | Amount in Dollars |
|---|---|
| Tuition and fees (1/12 of annual) | _____ |
| Textbooks and supplies (1/12 of annual) | _____ |
| Housing: monthly mortgage, rent, or room and board | _____ |
| Home repairs (estimated) | _____ |
| Renter's insurance (1/12 of annual) | _____ |
| Property tax (1/12 of annual) | _____ |
| Average monthly utilities (electricity, water, gas, oil) | _____ |
| Optional utilities (cell phone, Internet service, cable TV) | _____ |
| Dependent care, babysitting | _____ |
| Child support, alimony | _____ |
| Groceries | _____ |
| Meals and snacks out (including coffee, water, etc.) | _____ |
| Personal expenses (toiletries, cosmetics, haircuts, etc.) | _____ |
| Auto expenses (payments, gas, tolls) plus 1/12 of annual insurance premium—or public transportation costs | _____ |
| Loan repayments, credit card pay-off payments | _____ |
| Health insurance (1/12 of annual) | _____ |
| Prescriptions, medical expenses | _____ |
| Entertainment (movies, concerts, nightlife, sporting events, purchases of CDs, DVDs, video games, etc.) | _____ |
| Bank account fees, ATM withdrawal fees, credit card finance charges | _____ |
| Newspaper, magazine subscriptions | _____ |
| Travel, day trips | _____ |
| Cigarettes, smokeless tobacco | _____ |
| Beer, wine, liquor | _____ |
| Gifts | _____ |
| Hobbies | _____ |
| Major purchases (computer, home furnishings) (1/12 of annual) | _____ |
| Clothing, dry cleaning | _____ |
| Memberships (health clubs, etc.) | _____ |
| Pet food, veterinary bills, etc. | _____ |
| Other expenditure: _____ | _____ |
| Other expenditure: _____ | _____ |
| Other expenditure: _____ | _____ |
| Other expenditure: _____ | _____ |
| Other expenditure: _____ | _____ |
| **Total Monthly Outgoing** | _____ |

## School Loans, Grants, and More

Most schools offer financial aid. The federal government also offers several different types of aid. According to the U.S. Department of Education, more than nine million students receive some form of financial aid every year. This may include:

- *Flexible payment plans.* Some schools allow students to make several smaller payments throughout the semester instead of paying one lump sum for tuition expenses.

- *Loans.* A loan is an amount of money given by a lender. Loans must be repaid within a certain period of time, usually with interest. The federal government, as well as private lenders (banks), offer several different types of student loans.

- *Grants and scholarships.* Unlike loans, grants and scholarships do not have to be paid back. The qualifications are often highly specific. There may be a grant or scholarship out there just for you.

- *Work-study programs.* Some schools participate in work-study programs by arranging part-time jobs for students with financial need. Students are paid an hourly rate to earn money for tuition.

> *Questions about financial aid? Your financial aid advisor has answers!*

Financial aid is available to most students—take advantage of it! Make an appointment with one of your school's financial aid advisors. An advisor can help determine which type of aid will work best for you. But note: never take out more loans than you really need for your education. You don't want to spend the first 10 years of your new career struggling to pay them off!

## CHAPTER SUMMARY

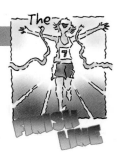

- Control stress by setting priorities, simplifying your life, learning to relax, thinking positively, and maintaining social supports.

- Regular exercise, good nutrition for physical and mental health, and plenty of sleep every night promote good health, reduce the risks of disease, and make it easier to succeed in school.

- Balance your school life with a social life that can contribute much to your well-being.

- Ensure you take steps to maintain your personal safety on and off campus.

- Use your personal budget to keep control over your finances and prevent debt that could stall your academic progress.

## REVIEW QUESTIONS

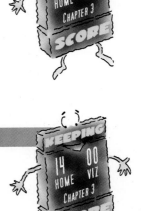

1. List three specific stress reduction techniques that work for you as an individual.

2. Name four foods you will try to eat more of to improve your health and three dietary substances you will try to minimize in your meals.

3. Describe the benefits of regular exercise.

4. What kinds of unnecessary expenditures do you sometimes make that negatively affect your budget?

## CHAPTER ACTIVITIES

1. Go to www.mypyramid.gov and read about how to stay within your daily calorie needs in order to maintain an appropriate weight.

2. For further information on types of financial aid, visit the U.S. Department of Education website: www2.ed.gov/fund/grants-college.html

3. First complete the "Where Does the Money Go?" exercise in this chapter. Then get together with a friend and compare notes. Brainstorm together how you might change your habits to cut back in some areas to help minimize your debt.

## CHAPTER 4

# Interacting with Others

## WINNING STRATEGY

***On completion of this chapter and the learning activities you will be able to:***

- Know why it's important to get to know your instructors
- Describe how participating in class contributes to your success as a student
- List the benefits of networking with other students
- Participate in campus life
- Understand and celebrate diversity

Succeeding in school involves so much more than simply sitting in classes, reading textbooks and doing homework, and completing assignments and tests. Education is an active learning process and students learn best through interacting with their instructors and other students. This experience includes individual interactions with your instructor, participating in classes by engaging in discussions with the instructor and other students, and networking with other students outside class. This chapter explains how to create a network that can benefit your studies while helping you share what you've learned with others. People in your network can be great resources of information, advice, and support. As you meet more and more people through all your educational experiences, you are also learning more about cultural diversity and gaining skills that will also serve you well in your future health care career.

## GETTING TO KNOW YOUR INSTRUCTORS

From the first day of class on, you are getting to know your instructors. At the start you may have wondered what your instructors will be like. Will they be nice? Are they going to be fair? Will they present things so you can understand them? Are you going to like and respect them? Are they going to like and respect you? As you listen and observe in class from the first day, you will begin to pick up on the instructor's personality, communication style, and perception of students.

Getting to know your instructors helps put you ahead of the game because you'll feel comfortable in the classroom more quickly. In turn, you will be able to concentrate on your studies sooner and more effectively.

## Teaching Styles

Some instructors like to share their philosophies about teaching. They'll also let you know how they prefer to run their classes.

- Some instructors like a formal atmosphere where they lecture and students raise their hands during a specified question and answer period.

- Others prefer a more informal environment where there's open classroom discussion and students can interrupt at any time to ask questions.

Knowing your instructor's teaching style gives you an advantage in the classroom. You'll learn to anticipate your instructor's next moves. This will help you study for exams, take effective notes, and participate in class. The sooner you can do these things, the easier it will be to do well in the course.

## Making a Good Impression

Getting to know your instructors involves more than simply observing them. Keep in mind that they are observing you too! You are making an impression whether you want to or not. It's worthwhile to make a good impression from the start by being attentive in class, participating in class discussions, and not hesitating to interact with the instructor.

An important first step is to introduce yourself to the instructor early in the term, even on the first day of class. Although it may seem intimidating, this is a very important step toward becoming a successful student.

Be reassured—most instructors welcome opportunities to meet their students. They enjoy teaching and they like to get to know their students. As soon as the instructor learns your name and knows that you're serious about being successful, then you're one step ahead of hundreds of other students. This isn't brownnosing. It's just good strategy.

## YOU DON'T KNOW ME, BUT . . .

"You don't know me, but . . ." may be the first words that come to mind. But that phrase sounds self-doubting. Instead, practice an introduction that conveys confidence. Try saying something such as, "Hi, my name is Melody Harris. I'm taking this course as a prerequisite for my Radiology Technician Certification. I'm really looking forward to a great semester. I'll see you at the next class." It's as simple as that.

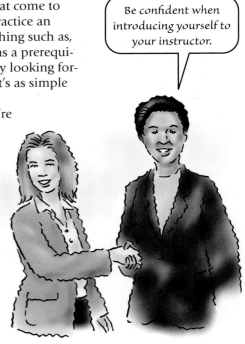

Be confident when introducing yourself to your instructor.

It's a good idea to plan ahead and practice what you're going to say. If you're especially anxious about this introduction, you might want to write down what you'd like to say and memorize it beforehand. When you approach the instructor, relax by taking a slow, deep breath. Then, put on a friendly smile, make eye contact, and make your introduction. If you're comfortable offering a handshake, that would be appropriate, too.

If your instructor didn't cover it in the class introduction in the first class, now is an ideal time to ask about the best way to contact him or her when needed. Should you have any questions over the course of the semester, you'll need to know how to get in touch with your instructor. Some instructors prefer email. Others prefer a visit during their office hours or a phone call. Be sure to make a note of this information.

## CLOSE ENCOUNTERS

There are places, such as large lecture halls that hold hundreds of students, where it may not be possible to introduce yourself after class. In these cases, consider seeking out the instructor during office hours to make your introduction. Your instructor certainly will remember and be impressed with you. And, in this more relaxed setting, the instructor may engage you in conversation for a few minutes about your career plans or the class. You may walk away with some interesting insights and valuable information.

## Instructor Conferences

It's a good idea to have an individual conference with every instructor at least once during the semester or term. A student-teacher conference gives you the opportunity to ask questions about lecture content, learn about your instructor's expectations of students, or discuss any other important issues related to the course.

Here are a few tips to consider when scheduling a conference:

- Decide on a specific topic to discuss, such as your first test or a confusing concept from a recent lecture.
- Write down any questions you'd like to ask about that topic, putting your most important questions at the top of the list. Your instructor may have a limited amount of time to meet with you.

> Schedule a student–teacher conference to learn more about what your instructor expects of students.

If you're organized and prepared for the meeting, you'll have a better chance of getting the information you need in that short period of time. Also, if the idea of a student–teacher conference makes you nervous, having questions already written out will put your mind at ease and help you stay focused.

By taking initiative and meeting with your instructor one-on-one, you'll demonstrate that you're concerned about your success as a student. You'll also gain a better understanding of your instructor. This will help you make sure you're on the same wavelength—it's always better to be aware of your instructor's expectations than to blindly assume you're doing well in a course.

## PARTICIPATING IN CLASS

Participating in class, interacting with the instructor and other students as part of the group, is also essential for being actively engaged in learning. Those who fail to participate, who sit passively in the classroom listening to others, are not fully engaged. They simply will not learn as well as those who make the effort to speak up. This principle applies both in lecture and discussion classes as well as laboratory classes.

### A Winning Game Plan

How can you pave the way for success in the classroom? There are several tactics you can use to join in and participate:

- Sit in the front of the room.
- Make sure you can see projection screens and in-class demonstrations.
- Make sure you can hear your instructor clearly.

- Ask questions to the instructor when appropriate.
- Answer questions the instructor asks the class.
- Respond to the comments of other students when invited by the instructor.

## But Why Participate?

Remember that education is an *active* experience. You don't just passively receive knowledge and skills by sitting there like a stone. Participating in class is the best way to actively engage. Here are some of the benefits of participating:

- Studies show that students actively engaged by participating in class learn more—and thus get better grades. One reason is that when you speak out in class and answer instructors' questions, you are more likely to remember the discussion than if you were passively listening to others speak.

- Paying close attention, thinking critically about what an instructor is saying, and making an effort to relate what is being said in a lecture can dramatically improve your enjoyment of the class and your impression of the instructor. You'll notice things you'll miss if you're feeling bored. You also may discover your instructor is much more interesting than you first thought.

- Asking the instructor questions, answering the instructor's questions posed to the class, and responding to other students' comments is a good way to make a good impression on your instructor. Then, in office hour visits and other interactions, the instructor will remember you as an engaged student. This helps you form an effective relationship with the instructor if you later need extra help or maybe even a mentor.

- Participating in class discussions is also a good way to start meeting other students. You may meet others with whom you can form a study group, borrow class notes if you miss a class, or team up with in a group project. Other students are often happy when you ask a question that was in their mind too and you'll gain their respect and find it easier to talk with them outside class.

> Take a step toward success by being a front-runner. Sit in the front row on the first day of class!

# The Front-Runner

Most of us have been to school assemblies or conferences where there are rows of seats. The front of the room is where the speaker's chair or podium is placed. As everyone files in to choose their seats, not many people go straight to the front row to sit. Even when there is "standing room only," seats in the front row often stay empty. We could spend a lot of time analyzing this scenario, but let's cut to the chase: sitting up front in the classroom is actually a very good thing.

Often students would rather blend into the background. They don't want to be noticed by the instructor or other students. Although you may have serious reservations about sitting in the front of the classroom, you'll find that it's in your best interest. Just remember—you're the student with the winning game plan. You're the one who's going to slide into home plate with room to spare.

If you think only the "A" students sit up front, you may be right. But they probably became "A" students by choosing to sit up front, in addition to employing other strategies. It takes effort to achieve success in the classroom. Sitting in the front row is one way to demonstrate that you're willing to make the effort. It also makes it easier to interact with the instructor during the class.

## TURN UP THE VOLUME

When choosing a seat up front, be sure to find one that lets you hear the instructor well. If you miss hearing important information in any class, it can have a negative effect on your overall performance in the course.

## THE ROAR OF THE CROWD

Classrooms tend to get noisy. One example is when the instructor discusses clinical rotation assignments. This is a very exciting time in health professions classes. Often, before the instructor can finish explaining all the details, students start talking back and forth. Some students begin asking the instructor questions while other students continue talking among themselves. The noise level rises. Unfortunately, this is when students either completely miss what the instructor is saying or hear it incorrectly. Misinformation then gets passed from student to student.

By sitting near the instructor, however, you'll be more likely to hear over the noise. When you're able to hear clearly, you can be one of the informed students who leaves class knowing exactly when and where you are supposed to go for your clinical assignment.

## "How Do I Do It?"

If you're one of those students who has always sat quietly in class, you may have to take active steps to start participating. Following are some pointers to get going.

When your instructor asks a question to the class:

- Raise your hand and make eye contact, but don't wave your hand all around trying to catch attention or call out. This isn't a game where the first, wildest, or loudest one wins!

- Be sure you have something to say before speaking. Take a moment to gather your thoughts and take a deep breath. Don't just blurt it out, but speak calmly and clearly.

When you want to ask the instructor a question:

- Don't ever feel your question is "stupid." If you have been paying attention in class and have done the reading and you still don't understand something, you have every right to ask. Many others in the class are probably wondering the same thing too!

- Ask at the appropriate time. Even if the instructor has said you can ask a question at any time, don't try to interrupt the instructor mid-sentence. Wait for a natural pause and a good moment to ask. But, unless the instructor asks students to hold all questions until the end of class, don't let too much time go by or you may forget your question.

- Be sure it's a real question, not an admission that you weren't paying attention. If you drifted off during the first half of class, don't ask a question about something that was already covered.

- Be open minded and show you really do want to learn. Don't let your question sound like a complaint or disagreement. You may be thinking: "Why would so-and-so believe that? That's just crazy!" But take a moment to think about what you're feeling. It's much better to say, "I don't understand what so-and-so is saying here. What evidence did he/she use to argue for that position?"

- Be sensitive to the needs of other students and avoid dominating a discussion.

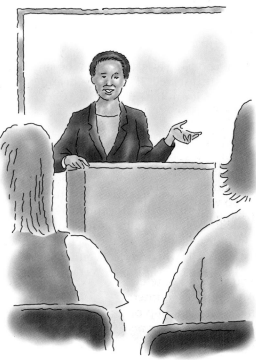

Remember, there's no such thing as a "stupid" question. But it can be "dumb" not to ask if you don't understand something!

When your instructor asks you a question directly:

- Be honest and admit it if you don't know the answer or are not sure. Don't try to fake it or make excuses. With a question that asks for an opinion, feel free to express your ideas openly. It's also fine to explain why you haven't decided yet.

- Organize your thoughts before answering. Instructors seldom want just a yes-or-no answer. Give your answer and then provide reasons for your position.

## Participation Helps Your Instructor Too

By staying engaged and asking questions about the lecture, you'll also help your instructor clear up any misunderstandings about the material. Other students might be confused about the same concepts that are confusing to you. The instructor's answers to your questions may be helpful to your classmates as well.

Also, by speaking up in class, you'll let your instructors know how well you're grasping the material they're presenting. When instructors feel that students are keeping up with the pace of the class, they know their teaching is being successful. If students are not keeping up, they can make adjustments or present the material in a different way.

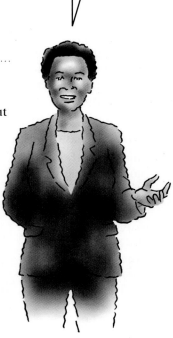

*Your network is your home team—it's easier to succeed when you work together!*

## NETWORKING WITH OTHER STUDENTS

Networking with other students is another key way to actively participate in your education. Networking should be an integral part of your winning strategy—not only while you're in school, but later on in your health care career. In school, your network is an informal academic support system that you develop with some of your classmates.

So what exactly is networking? How does it differ from simply having friends?

## The Home Team

You've heard of television networks and computer networks. A network is an interconnected group or system. A television network is a group of local stations that share the same programming. A computer network is a group of computers that share information. A network can be big or small.

A network also can be a group of people who choose to share information and expertise with one another. Usually, people "network" with others who share their interests or occupation. A network has several key features:

- It is voluntary—you choose to join and participate in a network.
- It is focused—information and expertise on a specific topic are shared.
- It is respectful—members all treat each other with respect, sharing ideas and asking questions freely.

Sometimes, a network forms naturally. For example, your instructor might put you into a group in class. You might find this group stays together even after the course is over. But usually, networks have to be purposely created.

## Why Network?

Networking is valuable for many reasons. Having a study group you can count on, getting tips for succeeding in a certain instructor's course, and being able to borrow notes from someone when you can't make it to class are all good reasons to network. As a student, networking gives you advantages you wouldn't have if you choose to keep to yourself.

Perhaps the most important reason to network is to give and receive support. Your peers at school probably understand better than anyone else the challenges you're facing. Members of your network can offer support by

*You're in the same boat as many of your classmates. Share what you know and learn from others by networking.*

- listening to your ideas
- sharing ideas with you
- making study time more relaxing
- helping you in tough times

Networks provide support by bringing people with the same goals together to help each other. The more you give, the more you get, and the better you feel.

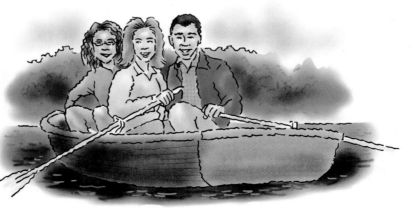

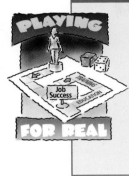

## Unexpected Benefits of Networking

Hi, my name is Roman and I'm training to become a medical coding specialist. I didn't like the idea of networking when I first started taking courses. It's hard for me to meet new people and I usually prefer to work on my own anyway.

But when I started having trouble in my medical terminology course, I had to ask for help. My academic advisor suggested that I talk to some of my classmates and try to form a study group. It wasn't easy, but I introduced myself to a couple of guys in my class and we started meeting regularly every week. Not only did my grades improve, but I ended up gaining two friends—something I wasn't expecting at all!

## Casting Your Net for an Informal Network

Even if you're shy or not very good at meeting new people, you'll find that informal networking is fairly simple and painless. Begin by introducing yourself to students sitting near you in class. If a conversation ensues, great! If not, you can speak to them again at the next class.

After you've spoken to another student a few times, bring up the idea that the two of you could make a deal. Propose that the two of you periodically share or compare lecture notes. Mention that you think it might help both of you understand the material better if you go over your notes together. You also can offer to share your notes if your classmate ever has to miss a lecture. If you're willing to help someone else, that person may be willing to share information with you when you need it.

Because everyone's schedules are already full, it may be difficult to arrange a time to meet. You might suggest meeting in the campus library or student study lounge a few minutes before class once a week. Your new acquaintances might not take you up on your offer right away. If they don't like the idea of networking, they may not realize they're turning down an excellent opportunity. If the first student you talk to is not interested, don't take it personally. Just move on, meet other classmates, and try again.

## Creating a More Formal Network

Creating a more formal network requires three things:

- You have a reason for forming the network. That way, you can keep the network focused. The reason may be to form a study group, for example. This study technique is discussed in more detail in Chapter 8.

- You add value to the network. You can contribute information as well as consume it.
- You have ground rules for participation.

Creating a network takes time, but it's worth it. If you develop a network of people you know and like, who can help you *and* learn from you, then you'll get the full benefit of this kind of interaction. Learning how to network successfully is very important for your future career, when you'll need to keep up on the latest information and techniques.

### FIRST-ROUND DRAFT PICKS

Begin by making a list of some classmates you'd like to include in your network. Choose two or three people from that list. Your network can grow over time, but it's best to start small. You'll find it's easier with a small group to get to know everyone and to arrange times to meet.

To narrow your list, think about the people on it:

- How much time does each person have to spend?
- How might each person contribute?
- What are people's strengths and weaknesses?
- Have you ever worked together before?

Weaknesses don't necessarily disqualify someone—we all have them. But think about how that person will fit into the group.

### SETTING UP THE RULES

Once you have your list, approach the people on it and suggest networking. The key here is to be clear about what you're proposing and to be respectful. If you want to have an informal network, where members email when they have a question or something to contribute, explain that. If you want a formal network, where members meet regularly in addition to emailing and having one-on-one conversations, make that clear.

Remember to be open to the suggestions and constraints of others. If someone can't meet when you'd like but is very valuable to the network, be flexible so you can include them. If someone doesn't have the time or simply doesn't want to be part of a formal network, graciously thank them and let them off the hook. That student can still be a personal, one-on-one source of information and sharing for you.

## Using Your Network

Remember, networking means interaction. Everyone in the network contributes information *and* consumes it. That's what makes the network valuable; everyone benefits from everyone else's knowledge and different ways of looking at things. When you network, you share what you know with others who do the same, creating something new in the combination of ideas. It's the sharing of ideas, or the dialogue, that makes a network successful.

## GIVE CREDIT WHERE CREDIT IS DUE

Information shared in a network is free. If something is shared in a network, all the members of the network should be allowed to use the information. But that doesn't mean you write down what someone else says and pass it off as your own opinion or knowledge. Always acknowledge your network. Be honest by saying your idea was inspired by someone in your network.

Be safe! Only give out your email address and phone number to people you trust. And **never** share other people's contact information without asking first!

## STAY SAFE

Once your networking group is established, you're likely to have people's phone numbers and other personal information, like email addresses or home addresses. Guard these carefully and don't share them with anyone without asking first. And remember not to wear out your network with constant contact, especially with network members who are busy with their home lives and jobs.

# When to Network

Informal networking goes on all the time—between classes, over lunch, and on the phone. Activate your formal network at specific times:

- *At the beginning of the semester.* Find out which students in your class have had this instructor before and what you should expect. Ask them for tips and advice about being successful in this class, but *never* ask for old tests and quizzes.

- *After class or lab sessions.* Strike while the iron is hot. Talk about the ideas you had during class, find out what your classmates thought, and then debate and expand the conversation. Take notes of your conversations next to your lecture notes.

- *After a missed class.* Call on your network to fill you in, but remember not to lean on your network to do your work for you.

## Network Online

You also can network online. This works well for a network that is spread out. For instance, if your cousin is a health professional in another state, you can include him or her in an online network. Just remember to be careful online. All the rules for face-to-face networks apply here. Only talk online with people you trust and don't invite strangers in without talking with the whole group first. Avoid giving out network members' email addresses. You should only share information online with people you know and trust.

# ACADEMIC ADVISORS AND COUNSELORS

So far in this chapter, we've discussed the many benefits of interacting with both instructors and other students—and the value this has for your academic success and future career. But there are others, too, on campus with whom your interaction is very important, including those in administrative and counseling offices. Among these, the most important for students are academic advisors.

## They're Here to Help

A school's academic counselors are there to advise students. Counselors work with course catalogs and student problems every day. If you have a question about your requirements, or if you just need advice, your school's academic counselors are great resources. They can often provide you with information you won't find in the course catalog.

It's also important to establish a relationship with your academic counselors for the future. Some schools offer job placement services as well. Your school's academic counselors may be important contacts to have in your network once you begin looking for a full-time position in your field.

# CAMPUS LIFE

The social world of your school is an important part of the total experience. Social relationships help make you feel more at home on campus and also contribute to your happiness and success as a student. Take advantage of opportunities to meet new people and become involved in campus life.

- Keep the door open for meeting new people. For example, don't follow the same routine with your meals on campus, but try to sit with different people so you can get to know them in a relaxed setting. Study in a common area or lounge where others may happen upon you when you need to take a break or study with someone else.

- Stay open in your interests. Don't limit yourself just to past interests, or you'll miss many opportunities to make friendships that may start based on some other activity.

- On the other hand, don't try to get involved in everything going on around you. Overcommitting yourself to too many activities or trying to join too many social groups will spread yourself too thin. Remember: it's the quality, not the quantity, of your social interactions that matters.

- Let others see who you really are. How can someone want to spend time interacting with you if they don't know who you are?

- While letting others get to know you, make an effort to get to know them, too. Show some interest. Don't talk just about your interests—ask them about theirs. Show others that you're interested, that you think they're worth spending time with, that you really do want to get to know them. It's easy enough to show your feelings with casual comments like, "It was really fun studying together—I think we should do it again!"

- Once a friendship has started, be a good friend. Respect your friend for what he or she is and don't criticize them or talk about them behind their back. Take the time to understand your friend when they're feeling sad or frustrated or just "need a friend." Give emotional support when your friend needs it and accept their support as well when you need it.

## Clubs and Organizations

Organized groups and activities offer a great way to enrich your social interactions on campus. But participating in organized activities requires some initiative—you can't be passive and expect these opportunities to come knocking on your door. A stimulating life on campus offers many benefits, including these:

- Organized groups and activities speed your transition into your new life as a student.

- Organized groups and activities help you experience a much greater variety of social life. If you interact only with other students your own age with similar backgrounds, you'll miss out on the broader campus diversity: students who are older and may have a perspective you may otherwise miss, upperclass students who can share much from their experience, and students of diverse heritage or culture whom you might not meet otherwise.

- Organized groups and activities help you gain new skills, whether technical, physical, intellectual, or social. Such skills may find their way into your résumé when you next seek a job or your application for a scholarship or other future educational opportunity. Employers like to see well-rounded students with a range of proficiencies and experiences.

- Organized groups and activities are fun and a great way to relieve to stay healthy and stress. As discussed in Chapter 2, exercise and physical activity are essential for health and well-being and many organized activities offer a good way to keep moving.

## FINDING ACTIVITIES YOU LIKE

There are many ways to learn about groups on your campus and opportunities for various activities. Start by browsing the school's website, where you're likely to find links to student clubs and organizations. Watch for club fairs, open houses, and similar activities on campus. Especially near the beginning of the year, an activity fair may include tables set up by many groups to provide students with information. Look for notices on bulletin boards around campus. Stop by the appropriate school office, such as the student affairs or student activities office or cultural center. Most schools make an attempt to provide information about all clubs and groups on campus.

# DIVERSITY

Ours is a very diverse society—and increasingly so. Already in many parts of the country, non-Hispanic whites comprise more than 50% of the population and, by 2020, one in three Americans, and about half of all college students, will be a person of color. But "diversity" means much more than racial and ethnic differences. Diversity refers to the great variety of human characteristics—ways that we are different even as we are all human and share more similarities than differences. These differences enrich humanity and all of us as individuals.

Experiencing diversity while in school brings many benefits both in the present and for the future:

- Experiencing diversity in school prepares students for the diversity they will encounter the rest of their lives. Those who work in health care careers will work with other professionals and patients who may be very different from themselves. Success in your future career will require being able to understand people in new ways and interacting with new skills. Experiencing diversity in school assists in this process.

- Students learn better in a diverse educational setting. Encountering new concepts, values, and behaviors leads to thinking in deeper, more complex, more creative ways. Studies have shown, for example, that students who experience racial and ethnic diversity in their classes are more engaged in active thinking processes and develop more intellectual and academic skills than others with limited experience of diversity.

- Experiencing diversity on campus is beneficial for both minority and majority students. All students have more fulfilling social relationships and report more satisfaction and involvement with their academic experience.

- Diversity experiences help break patterns of segregation and prejudice that have characterized American history. Discrimination against others—whether by race, gender, age, sexual orientation, or anything else—is rooted in ignorance and sometimes fear of people who are different. Getting to know people who are different is the first step in accepting those differences, furthering the goal of our society becoming free of all forms of prejudice and unfair treatment of people.

- Experiencing diversity makes us all better citizens in our democracy. When we can better understand and consider the ideas and perspectives of others, we are better equipped to participate meaningfully in our society. This is especially important for those in health care careers.

- Diversity enhances self-awareness. We gain insights into our own thought processes, life experiences, and values as we learn from people whose backgrounds and experiences are different from our own.

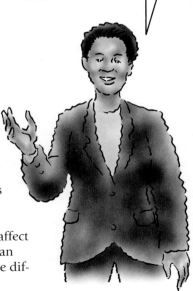

Part of being a professional means treating everyone you encounter—patients, supervisors, and coworkers—with equal care and respect.

## What Is Cultural Diversity?

When people talk about cultural diversity, they are referring to the ways in which all people are similar to and different from each other. Racial classifications, ethnicity, gender, sexual orientation, religious affiliation, socioeconomic status, and age are all elements of cultural diversity.

It's natural to note differences between yourself and those around you. As you enter the world of health care, it is important to understand that, regardless of differences, you must treat everyone with equal care and respect. This means refusing to allow any preconceived notions about others to affect the quality of your work. By openly accepting diversity, we can move closer toward appreciating the things that make people different and treating everyone with the same care and respect.

Cultural diversity is an especially important part of health care because of the genetic characteristics, cultural values, and belief systems that affect people's health. By knowing and understanding these cultural differences, you'll be able to provide better care.

## RACE AND ETHNICITY

The term *race* is typically based on a person's physical characteristics, such as skin color, facial features, hair texture, and body stature. *Ethnicity* is the concept of identifying with the traditions and values of a particular cultural group. Although the terms ethnicity and race are often used interchangeably, they refer to different aspects of a person's identity. An individual can be of one race, yet identify with a different ethnicity.

In health care, race is sometimes a factor in diagnosis and treatment because genetic traits are often more common in certain racial groups than in others. Likewise, ethnic values and traditions also can have an effect on a patient's health and well-being.

## GENDER ROLES

It's important to consider gender roles when interacting with others of a different background. In some cultures, for example, the male is considered the head of the household. In these cases, a male family member might speak for his female family members. In other cultures, women are the dominant family members. It's important that health care professionals consider this when providing care. Gender roles may influence the way in which a patient prefers to be treated. Every patient has a different role in the family and it's important to be sensitive to the different needs and priorities of each.

## SEXUAL ORIENTATION

A person's sexual orientation is a personal matter—true for both your fellow students and patients and coworkers with whom you will interact in the future. Again, it is important not to prejudge another person but to accept all forms of diversity. In health care, there are times when sexual orientation may be an important issue, such as when addressing sexually transmitted diseases. Regardless of what information patients choose to reveal, it's important to avoid making judgments or assumptions about a patient's sexual orientation or lifestyle choices.

## RELIGION

Everyone has freedom of religion in our society and all people's religious choices should be respected. In health care, patients' religious beliefs and values may affect how they wish to be treated by health care professionals. For example, a person's religious affiliation can influence decisions about diet and nutrition, sexual lifestyle, and other health matters. As a health care professional, you'll need to be sensitive to each patient's values and beliefs when providing care. You can do this by respecting the personal choices made by patients and adapting care to suit each patient's needs.

## Keeping an Open Mind

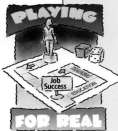

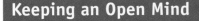

My name is Ling and I'm a medical assistant. There was one patient I came across during my clinical experience who I thought had something against women. He wouldn't let me take his blood pressure—he always asked for a man to do it. I thought he was prejudiced against me and, I admit, I felt angry. So I talked to my mentor. She told me that I shouldn't make assumptions or take his actions personally. She said that part of providing the best care meant doing what I could to accommodate different patients' needs, whether they make sense to me or not.

Later, I found out that the patient was an Orthodox Jew and it was against his religion to be touched by a woman not in his family. I was embarrassed about my assumptions. After that, I made sure a male medical assistant was around to take the patient's blood pressure and other vital signs during his office visits.

## SOCIOECONOMIC STATUS

Socioeconomic status is yet another way in which people are different and no one should be judged or discriminated against based on such differences. A person's socioeconomic status should not affect the kind of care and treatment that a health care professional provides. Every patient, regardless of financial situation, should be given the best possible care and attention. Avoid stereotyping patients according to their level of education or how much money they make. Instead, focus on each patient as an individual worthy of your attention, respect, and sensitivity.

## AGE

Age is another of the many ways in which individuals differ. In health care, age is often important because the aging process affects the health of patients in different ways. Younger patients often have health care needs different from those of older patients. You'll need to be sensitive to patients' changing physical and emotional needs as they grow older. It's also essential that you avoid making assumptions about a patient based on age. It is important to remember that physical fitness and health can vary for different people at every age and stage in their lives.

## Celebrate Diversity!

Diversity is not something just to know in your head like a concept you've learned in school. Diversity is an essential part of the rich experience of humanity—it is something to be celebrated and embraced as part of being human! Don't think of diversity as something to be aware of just in your future health care profession as you work with patients. You'll grow as a person as you seek out diverse experiences now as a student and actively promote understanding of the many differences among us all.

Here are things you can do to celebrate diversity, challenge old stereotypes, and promote a healthy multiculturalism on your campus and in your community:

- Acknowledge your own uniqueness, for you too are diverse.
- Consider your own (possibly unconscious) stereotypes so you can work to eliminate them.
- Do not try to ignore differences among people.
- Do not expect all individuals within any group to be alike.
- Don't apply any group generalizations to individuals.
- Take advantage of campus opportunities to increase your cultural awareness, such as cultural fairs and celebrations, concerts, and other programs.
- Take the initiative in social interactions with diverse others.
- Work through any conflicts as in any other social interaction.
- Take a stand against prejudice and hate when you see it.

### CHAPTER SUMMARY

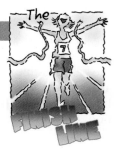

- Make a good first impression on your instructors. Introduce yourself and plan a visit for an individual conference during office hours.
- Sit in the front of the room. Have a great seat with the best view and best sound. This sets you up for successful participation in class.
- Ask questions in class and answer those posed by your instructors. Active engagement in the process is the most effective way to learn.
- Network with other students to get ahead. Develop good study networks that will help you learn and support your academic goals. Remember to play it safe.
- Networking is important because it allows you to share your ideas and learn from others. Networks also can be a source of support during the challenges you face as a student.

- Investigate campus organizations and activities to become part of the wider academic community while having fun and maintaining your health.
- Challenge yourself to better understand and celebrate the diverse differences among people. Never prejudge others who are different from you in any way.

## REVIEW QUESTIONS

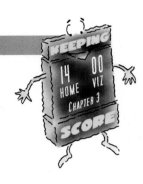

1. Why is it important to sit in the front of the classroom?
2. What is an example of a time when health professions classrooms become particularly noisy? Why is it essential to be able to hear your instructor at a time like this?
3. Give an example of how you might be making an impression on your instructors even when you may not be aware of it.
4. How would introducing yourself to your instructor help prepare you for future clinical experience?
5. List several benefits of developing both an informal and formal network with other students.
6. What are several challenges you might face when creating a network?
7. List at least six ways in which people may be different from each other.
8. Why should diversity be celebrated?

## CHAPTER ACTIVITIES

1. Networking Exercise: Talk with at least two friends at school about creating a network. Each of you will then come up with one other person you know and trust from one of your classes. Give yourselves a week to contact the other people. Then, meet as a group to see how you all get along. If everyone seems like compatible network members, decide on a place and time to meet regularly.
2. Campus Life Activity: Using the tips presented in this chapter to learn about campus organizations and activities at your school, find at least three you might be interested in participating in. Using the school's website or other resources, investigate these three to learn more about what goes on in each.

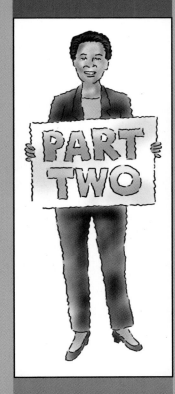

# SHARPENING YOUR SKILLS

## CHAPTER 5

# Making the Most of Your Learning Style

*On completion of this chapter and the learning activities you will be able to:*

- Describe the brain's role in learning

- Identify your learning style and know how to make the most of it

- Explain how critical thinking applies in health care settings

- Describe Benjamin Bloom's six levels of cognitive learning

Do you know there are different styles of learning? For example, you might absorb information better when you see it (as in a chart) than when you hear it (as in a lecture). Some people learn better when they can "do" the material, as in a lab experiment. Most classes are made up of students who have a variety of different learning styles. What works for one student might not work as well for the next.

This chapter discusses several major learning styles and how you can use your individual learning style, as well as other methods, to become a successful student. We'll also talk about the importance of critical thinking and how it relates to both learning and your future career.

## LEARNING STYLES

Your brain, and how it functions, is a contributing factor to the way you learn. By understanding how your brain works, you'll be on your way to understanding your particular learning style. And, by being aware of your learning style, you'll discover ways you can learn more efficiently.

# The Brain and Learning

The human brain weighs about three pounds. Although small, this organ functions as the control center for the entire body. It determines how a person thinks, feels, and acts. The brain is where all learning takes place.

## YOUR HARDWORKING BRAIN

It's true that people use only a percentage of the brain's full capability. Even so, the human brain is responsible for an amazing number of functions, including:

- breathing, circulation, temperature regulation, and other involuntary functions
- balance and equilibrium
- voluntary actions
- emotional reactions
- reasoning and thinking
- the ability to convert things you experience with your senses into recognizable images, sounds, feelings, smells, or tastes

## BRAIN ZONES

The three main areas of the brain include:

- the brain stem
- the cerebellum
- the cerebrum (see *The Human Brain*)

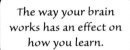

The way your brain works has an effect on how you learn.

---

**The Human Brain**

The three main areas of the brain all have different roles in the learning process:

- Brain stem: connects the brain to the spinal cord and controls basic functions
- Cerebellum: controls basic functions such as balance and coordination
- Cerebral cortex: controls high-level functions and voluntary muscle movements

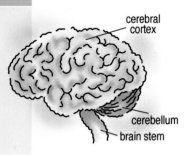

cerebral cortex

cerebellum

brain stem

---

## *Star Players: The Brain Stem and Cerebellum*

The different areas of the brain all work together. However, each area is responsible for controlling certain functions. For example, the brain stem and cerebellum, located nearest the spinal cord, control basic functions. These areas of your brain determine your body's ability to maintain muscle tone. They also regulate involuntary actions, such as your heartbeat and breathing.

*Team Captain: The Cerebrum*

The cerebrum, the largest portion of the brain, contains the cerebral cortex. The cerebral cortex is very complex. It controls many high-level functions of the mind, such as sight and conscious thought. It also controls the body's voluntary muscle movements.

The brain's cortex is divided into two hemispheres. Different types of thought processes begin in each hemisphere:

- The left hemisphere is responsible for controlling language and logical thinking. In terms of physical movement, the left hemisphere controls the right side of the body.

- The right hemisphere controls nonverbal processes, such as intuitive thinking and imagination. It manages movement of the left side of the body.

You may have heard the expressions "left-brained" and "right-brained." A person who is an artistic daydreamer may be considered "right-brained." A mathematician, on the other hand, may be considered "left-brained." One hemisphere of their brains may be more dominant, making certain tasks easier than others. This doesn't mean those individuals only use a single hemisphere of their brains. On the contrary, the left and right hemispheres of the brain are always active in everyone. Whether your personality is more logical or creative, you can use both sides of your brain. When it comes to learning, knowing your brain's strengths and weaknesses is helpful.

---

**Left Brain vs. Right Brain**

You may be a musician with an ear for rhythm or a math whiz with an eye for sequential order. In either case, both hemispheres of your brain are available to help you learn. By recognizing which hemisphere of your brain is stronger, you'll become aware of the kinds of tasks that require your brain to work slightly harder. The illustration on the right lists the major "left-brain" and "right-brain" reasoning tasks.

Left Hemisphere
- language and word use
- logic, reason, and analysis
- numbers and math
- rational thought
- sequence and order

Right Hemisphere
- artistic perception
- creativity
- intuitive thought
- music and rhythm
- imagination and abstract thought
- daydreaming and reflection
- random thought

---

## ON A CELLULAR LEVEL

There are two main types of brain cells:

- *glial cells.* These cells are the brain's supporting structures.
- *neurons.* These cells receive and send messages to one another in the form of electrochemical nerve impulses. Neurons play a role in complex functions of the mind and body, such as learning, motion, and sensations.

## Good News Travels Fast!

News travels fast in the human brain. For example, an electrical signal travels from one neuron to the next at a rate of 200 miles per hour (100 meters per second)! These electric signals move from one neuron to another through a network of dendrites and axons.

The following steps trace the path of an electrical signal from one neuron to the next:

1. The electrical signal travels down the axon.
2. The axon releases neurotransmitters (chemicals).
3. The neurotransmitters travel across the synaptic gap and are received by the dendrites of the next neuron.
4. The next neuron absorbs the neurotransmitters.
5. The neurotransmitters change the second neuron's electrical state.
6. A new electrical pulse is produced by the second neuron.

## Making Connections

Each infant is born with a complete set of neurons. As a child learns, those neurons develop connections between themselves. Every time sensory cells are stimulated by outside forces, nerve impulses travel from one neuron to the next.

Every time you learn something new, the neurons in your brain begin sending messages in a certain pattern. If stimulation is repeated, it becomes easier for the same nerve impulses to travel from one neuron to the next. This is because patterns begin to form and the neurons involved gain better connections between themselves. Your neurons "learn" these patterns and develop faster ways of communicating with each other.

*Learning new things, such as how to ride a bike, develops connections between your neurons. The more you practice something, the stronger those connections become.*

## Losing Ground

Learning new information causes the number of connections between your neurons to increase. Unfortunately, it's a two-way street. As soon as you stop learning new things, some of those connections begin to disappear. The solution to the problem is continued learning. You can rebuild those lost connections by relearning things you've forgotten.

## Keeping Your Brain Healthy

A healthy body translates to a healthy mind. By taking care of your body, you'll be taking care of your brain, too. And, if you treat your brain right, you'll become a better learner.

You're probably aware that your diet has an impact on your physical performance. A doughnut in the morning won't give you lasting energy. But a healthy breakfast, such as a bowl of oatmeal and a cup of yogurt, will give you energy. Believe it or not, the food you eat and the fluids you drink affect how you learn as well. Diet has been linked to mood, behavior, and mental performance. For example, substances called electrolytes actually speed your thought processes. These substances work as conductors in the brain. Electrolytes help conduct the electrical currents that travel from one neuron to the next. Put simply, they help your brain think faster and work more efficiently.

Chapter 3 discusses healthy eating as a way to help your body cope with stress. Another reason to have a well-balanced diet is that it can enhance your ability to learn.

## WHAT'S YOUR STYLE?

Now that we have looked at how the brain functions, let's focus on learning styles. A learning style is an individual's preferred way to receive and process information during the learning process. One student may learn better by reading about a topic, for example, whereas another student learns better by hearing the instructor talk about the topic.

Three major learning styles are:

- visual
- auditory
- kinesthetic

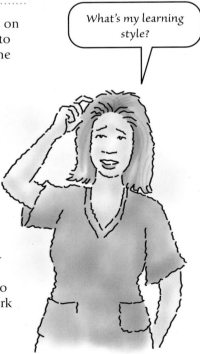

What's my learning style?

Just as one hemisphere of your brain might be more dominant than the other, it's likely that you prefer one particular learning style to the rest. There is no right or wrong style, no best or worst style—people simply learn in different ways. The key is to identify your own style and then use this knowledge to your advantage. Being aware of your learning strengths can help you improve your studying and test-taking skills. You'll also be better equipped to compensate for your weaknesses. By making your learning style work for you, you'll get more out of your courses. You'll have improved interaction with your instructors and other students. As an added benefit, you'll also more fully enjoy the learning process.

## The Eyes Have It

Visual learners prefer to read about things or watch demonstrations. They like looking at charts, diagrams, and images. They like it quiet when they study. They may use arrows and circles when taking notes to visually show relationships of ideas or their importance.

If you're a visual learner, seek out all kinds of visual materials. These include:

- textbooks
- demonstrations (in class or on video)
- handouts from your instructors
- information on the Internet
- lecture notes
- articles in magazines, newspapers, and professional journals

Here are some study tips for visual learners:

- Pay close attention to visual presentations.
- Take notes using visual cues (circles, arrows, color highlighting, concept maps).
- Highlight in your textbook and jot margin notes.
- Make flashcards that include visual cues to help you remember key concepts.
- When studying, visualize things the instructor wrote on the board or included in a PowerPoint presentation.

## Sounds Good to Me

Auditory learners gain the most information when they hear about things. This includes listening to your instructor and other students, as well as recorded presentations. If you learn best by listening, think of where you can find auditory information. Resources that may be helpful to you include:

- class discussions
- class lectures
- question-and-answer sessions
- giving speeches
- reading aloud
- recorded lectures or speeches (video or online)

Here are some study tips for auditory learners:

- Choose a class seat where you can hear well without noisy distractions.
- Form a study group with others who prefer to talk over course topics.

- Read your notes aloud when studying. Record your readings and replay.
- Record key class lectures (with instructor's permission) and review later as needed.
- Be sure to participate in class.

## Jump Right In

Kinesthetic learners prefer to learn by doing. They like to move around and may have difficulty sitting still for long periods. They prefer a hands-on approach to learning. If it's easier for you to grasp information after putting it to use by actively doing something, you're a kinesthetic learner. To enhance your learning opportunities:

- Seek out workshops and skills labs.
- Volunteer to perform in-class demonstrations.
- Attend field trips.
- Help out with group projects.
- Seek out internships or volunteer work in your field.
- Offer to tutor a classmate.

Here are some study tips for kinesthetic learners:

- Use interactive computer learning aids to engage with the subject.
- Study while physically moving; take frequent breaks to walk around; read assignments on a treadmill or exercise bike.
- Make flashcards frequently and sort them as you review.

### Being a Kinesthetic Learner

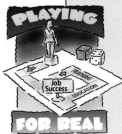

Hi, my name is Marcela and I'm training to become a surgical technician. I used to have a hard time learning new information. I'd read something and it wouldn't sink in. Or I'd sit and listen to a lecture only to feel like I wasn't getting it. I thought maybe I wasn't cut out for school.

That all changed when I took my first skills lab. All of a sudden, it's like a lightbulb went on in my head! When I had a chance to demonstrate my skills, I actually understood and remembered the procedures.

Now that I know I'm a kinesthetic learner, I look for other ways to help me learn, in addition to reading my textbooks and going to classes. I attend workshops, go on field trips, and get plenty of hands-on experience volunteering at a local hospital.

- If having difficulty sitting still, chew gum or repetitively tense and relax body muscles.
- Talk to a study partner while walking or jogging.

## Discovering Your Own Learning Style

From the preceding discussion, you probably already have a good idea about your own style. In reality, however, few people have purely only one learning style. You may favor one dominant approach, but likely you still learn through other styles also. To discover more exactly your preferences and receive tips to help you learn as fully as possible, take a few minutes to check out the learning styles assessment from MyPower Learning. You can access this by first visiting thePoint website that comes along with this text (http://thePoint.lww.com/StudentSuccess2e). See the inside front cover for login information. You can also visit the MyPower Learning website at www.mypowerlearning.com.

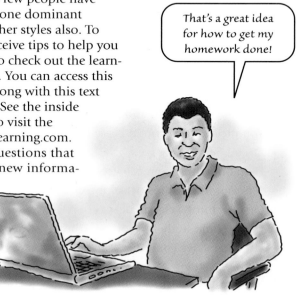

This learning style assessment asks you questions that relate to how you interact with and process new information. The questions are simple and easy to answer. Following the questions, you receive a custom report that evaluates your learning style preferences with comparative scores in the three styles described earlier: visual, auditory, and kinesthetic. Your scores identify your strongest style, your second strongest, and your least favored style.

Be sure to click on the "Detailed Report" option at the end of your score report and print it out for the list of tips for maximizing your learning in these three areas:

- Participating in class
- Doing homework assignments
- Preparing for class and exams

Students with different learning styles, or mixes of styles, will gain from different study and preparation techniques. It pays to find out what works best for you!

## How Large Do You Think?

Another difference in how people learn and think involves the scope of thought. Some people just naturally think in large, abstract terms—thinking globally. Others naturally think more in terms of the details. As with the previous learning styles, understanding your own thinking and learning preferences can help maximize your learning in classes.

> What do you usually see, the tree or the forest?

## GOING GLOBAL

Global learners excel when they think about the "big picture." If you're a global learner, you may find that you enjoy learning how concepts are related to one another. Your favorite instructor may be one who gives plenty of analogies to show how the information is connected. Or you may prefer a class where the instructor lays out certain facts and helps students make conclusions about the material. If this is the case, try using the following tips to get the most out of your courses:

- Summarize your lecture notes and draw conclusions about the material.

- Sketch diagrams to show how different ideas come together to form the "big picture."

- Come up with questions about the topics covered in class.

## IT'S ALL IN THE DETAILS

Detail learners prefer to learn new information in a logical pattern. For example, many people have had the experience of purchasing items labeled "some assembly required." If you're prone to looking at instruction manuals and following directions closely—as opposed to jumping right in and randomly trying to fit pieces together—you're probably a detail learner.

If you're a detail learner, you may do best in a class where the instructor follows a strict outline. But regardless of your instructor's teaching style, there are ways you can use your strengths to your advantage:

- Summarize your lecture notes with bulleted points.

- Draw diagrams to relate small pieces of information (details) to larger themes or ideas.

- Create a to-do list for yourself before you sit down to study.

- Write down questions as they come to mind during lectures or while reading.
- Think of examples you can use to illustrate particular details.

# CRITICAL THINKING AND LEARNING

Closely related to learning skills are critical thinking skills. It's especially important for health care professionals to have solid critical thinking skills. When you think critically, you analyze information to form judgments about it. The information may be gathered from your observations, personal experience, reasoning, or communication. In your profession, you may be required to gather and analyze information and evaluate results on a daily basis. If you're able to think critically and make good judgments based on the information you can gather, you'll have a positive impact on your patients' health.

## Critical Thinking Skills in the Workplace

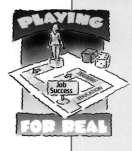

My name is Derek. I've been working as a certified medical assistant for about a year now and I've definitely had to put my critical thinking skills to the test! I work in a family practice office, so our patients are all ages and they come in for a lot of different reasons.

Last week, one of our patients made an appointment because he was experiencing abdominal pain. He arrived early for his appointment and said he was still experiencing pain and was feeling nauseous, too. I could tell he was in obvious distress—his skin was pale and he was holding his stomach in pain. Even though his appointment time wasn't for another 20 minutes, I decided to take him back to wait in an empty exam room. Then I gave the physician a heads-up about his symptoms, in case he needed to be examined right away. It's a good thing I did, because as it turned out, the patient had appendicitis!

## Direct Yourself to Learning

Individuals who are successful in both school and the workplace have achieved their success by becoming self-directed learners. Being a self-directed learner means that you take responsibility for your own education, regardless of your preferred learning style. In the coming chapters, you'll learn more about different ways to accomplish this.

For example, if you're having a hard time understanding a particular concept in class, you can find other resources, ask your instructor for clarification, or meet with your study group. Although test scores are important, your main goal in school should be to learn the material. Being a self-directed learner means not only studying in order to do well on tests and quizzes, but also studying in order to store information in your long-term memory. It also means being able to apply that information to new situations once you become a practicing health care professional.

Likewise, successful professionals must be self-directed learners. Once you are no longer a student, you'll have to take even more responsibility for your own learning. This may mean keeping yourself up-to-date on the latest research by reading articles related to your field. Or it may mean requesting to observe a procedure you've been struggling to learn. In these cases, you should be aware of what you need to learn and how you can go about increasing your knowledge and improving your skills.

Regardless of your past experience as a student, you can achieve success now by becoming a self-directed learner. You have chosen to further your education because of your motivation toward a particular career goal. Contrary to how you may feel at first, you *can* control a great deal of what you learn and how your educational experience will unfold.

Learning is a process. By understanding how the process works, you can begin to develop the learning skills you'll use as a student and later in your professional career.

> Learning is a process. You have to start at the bottom and work your way up to the next level.

## Bloom's Learning Levels

Cognitive learning, closely related to critical thinking, occurs in several stages. Benjamin Bloom, a noted neuropsychologist, assigned the following names to these stages in the 1950s:

- knowledge
- comprehension
- application
- analysis
- synthesis
- evaluation

Although other psychologists have developed new theories about thinking since the 1950s, most theories are similar to Bloom's. In other theories, the stages may be named or ordered differently, but their descriptions remain relatively the same.

## KNOWLEDGE

During the knowledge stage, you memorize information and repeat it word for word. At this point, you don't necessarily have to understand the information to memorize it. Some examples of things you may need to memorize are:

- formulas in a math class
- people's names, addresses, and phone numbers
- simple instructions, such as steps in a skill

## COMPREHENSION

In the comprehension stage, you understand information enough to be able to restate it in your own words. If you take effective notes during class, your notes should reflect your comprehension. You can accomplish this by:

- drawing charts and diagrams
- summarizing and paraphrasing information
- describing how concepts are related
- explaining the material to someone else

## APPLICATION

During this stage, you use the information you've memorized and comprehended to accomplish a task. Examples of application include:

- using a mathematical formula to solve a problem
- using a rule or principle to classify information
- successfully completing a project after receiving and following directions

## ANALYSIS

Analysis involves breaking information into parts to understand how those parts are organized and related to one another. For example, when you read an article in a magazine, you first look at the different pieces of information presented. An author may provide several anecdotes to illustrate a single main point. Then, you analyze the different pieces of information by thinking about how they are related. How does each anecdote relate to the author's theme or main point? What message is the author communicating?

## SYNTHESIS

In the synthesis stage, you put your analysis to use by developing a new idea. In a sense, you take parts of information and put them together in a different way to form a new concept. This stage of learning and thinking is more creative than the others. It includes:

- building on the pieces of information contained in your notes and writing a paper or presentation
- forming a plan for conducting a lab experiment
- writing a poem or short story

> Remember, critical thinking is a tool used not just by students, but by health care professionals as well.

### EVALUATION

During the last stage in critical thinking, you evaluate information. This means you use other methods, such as comprehension and analysis, to determine whether or not information has value or relevance. Evaluation can include:

- determining which conclusions are actually supported by facts and research
- judging the value of a work of art or a piece of writing based on specific standards
- determining the value and relevance of information presented in a textbook, lecture, or class discussion

## Be Critical

When reading your textbooks or other material, you shouldn't just passively receive the information but rather be an active reader. During active reading, it's important to be a critical reader. Now is the time to analyze the text and question the author. By asking questions about the text, you'll begin to think critically about the material. As a result, you'll improve your comprehension and remember more. You'll be better able to apply, analyze, and evaluate the information. Ask yourself:

- How would I apply this information if I were caring for a patient?
- How is this material related to what I've studied in the past?
- How does this information measure up to the information in other sources I've read? Does it support or contradict what I already know about the topic?
- Are there any inconsistencies?
- Does the author present an objective view of the material? Is the information based on assumptions, facts, experiences, or opinions?
- Do I agree with the author? Why or why not?
- On which topic would I like more information?

## CHAPTER SUMMARY

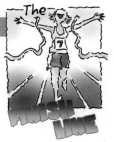

- Your brain plays a role in determining your particular learning style.
- Play to your strengths by identifying your learning style and being aware of how to enhance it.
- Enhance your learning and prepare for your future career by thinking critically about what you are learning.

## REVIEW QUESTIONS

1. Describe the benefits of knowing your own learning style preferences.
2. What types of resources or activities would be helpful to someone who is an auditory learner?
3. Write a definition for critical thinking in your own words.
4. Why do synthesis and evaluation learning skills come after knowledge and comprehension skills?

## CHAPTER ACTIVITIES

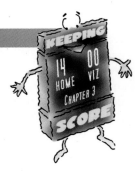

1. Discovering Your Learning Style: Take the learning styles assessment by My Power Learning by first visiting thePoint website (http://thePoint/lww.com/Student Success2e). Use the access code in the front cover of this textbook. After you take the assessment, print your Learning Style Index and specialized report.

2. Working Together: Divide into three groups based on your learning style assessment results (visual, auditory, or kinesthetic). In your group, come up with an idea for an activity or project that would help students with your learning style understand the information in this chapter. Then, write three to five sentences explaining how and why the activity or project would accommodate your particular learning style. Present your ideas to the other two groups in the class.

3. Critical Thinking Exercise: Review *Bloom's Learning Levels*. Draw a pyramid, set of stairs, skyscraper, or another image to illustrate Bloom's six levels of learning. Label each level and provide a practical example. For instance, a practical example for the lowest level of learning, knowledge, could be memorizing the definition of a key term and repeating it word for word.

## CHAPTER 6

# Listening, Taking Notes, and Reading

## WINNING STRATEGY

*On completion of this chapter and the learning activities you will be able to:*

- Use active listening techniques in the classroom
- Adjust to different lecture styles
- Maximize your learning in the classroom
- Take effective notes in class
- Develop a strategy for reading actively
- Create a note-taking outline

Listening, taking notes, and reading skills are all necessary if you want to succeed as a student. During lectures, it may seem like your only responsibility is to sit quietly while your instructor speaks. This method might even have served you well in high school. But now you have the opportunity to do much more! By using the strategies discussed in this chapter, you'll be able to take charge of your own learning process. And, when you're in control, nothing can stand in your way of learning new things and accomplishing your long-term goals. You'll be able to round the bases and slide safely into home!

## LISTENING SKILLS

The importance of listening carefully is discussed throughout this book. Good listening skills should be cultivated during your time in school. These skills will play a big role in your success not only as a student, but also as a health care professional. When miscommunication occurs in health care, the results can have negative consequences for patients.

Not hearing about assignments in school can, at the very least, result in frustration and grades that don't reflect your true ability.

A lot of valuable information is given out in class from the first day forward. Because most of it is verbal, it's worthwhile to start sharpening your listening skills. Make it a point to listen closely instead of jumping to conclusions. Watch and listen for essential clues in the classroom. Ask questions if you don't hear something and write down as much as you can to help you remember what was said.

*Give yourself a head start—practice good listening habits from day one in the classroom.*

## Active Listening

To become an active participant in your own learning process, try to keep your mind engaged instead of sitting back and relaxing while your instructor lectures. Make an effort to listen actively. To better understand the material, think of questions to ask the instructor. You can write your questions in your notes and refer back to them at the end of the lecture. If your instructor offers to answer questions toward the end of class, ask then. If not, look up the answers on your own after class.

There may be times, however, when you'll have a question that can't wait until the end of the lecture. If you feel that your instructor is moving too quickly, politely raise your hand and ask him or her to repeat or clarify a specific point. But keep in mind that you should do so only when you have prepared for the class properly beforehand—don't embarrass yourself by asking something you should already have known from doing assigned reading!

## Stop, Look, and Listen

Active listening involves thinking about how you are listening and continually working to improve your listening skills. When you are listening actively in the classroom, you're doing more than simply hearing words. You're also deciphering main ideas, deciding what information is most important, and making adjustments in how you listen according to your instructor's teaching style.

In the game of school, an active listener is participating in the game, not just standing on the sidelines. Whether you need to become an active listener or merely improve your active listening skills, all students can follow these guidelines:

- Avoid doing things that can distract you from listening.
- Identify main ideas.
- Pay attention to the speaker's transition cues.
- Mentally organize information as you hear it and devote your attention to material that seems more important.
- Take effective notes.

## INTERFERENCE!

There are several behaviors that could be sabotaging your active listening game. Make an effort to avoid:

- letting distractions interrupt your train of thought
- tuning out difficult material
- allowing your emotions to cloud your thinking
- assuming the material is boring
- concentrating on the speaker's quirks
- letting your mind wander
- pretending to listen
- listening only for facts and not ideas
- trying to write down every word in your notes

## IDENTIFY MAIN IDEAS

Identifying main ideas is a key element of active listening. Each lecture you hear will include main ideas even though they may be presented in different ways. Some of the approaches your instructor may take are:

- introducing new topics
- summarizing main points
- listing or discussing a main idea's supporting details
- showing two sides of the same issue
- discussing causes and effects related to a main idea
- identifying a main idea's problems and solutions

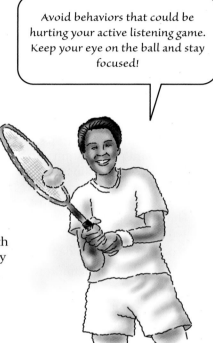

*Avoid behaviors that could be hurting your active listening game. Keep your eye on the ball and stay focused!*

## WAIT FOR A SIGNAL

Listening for signal words is another way to guide yourself through a lecture. These words are like play-by-play commentary in the classroom. They let you know which direction your instructor is headed.

Signal words can indicate transitions in a lecture. By paying attention to transitions, you'll be able to organize your thoughts and your notes as you listen actively. A few examples of signal words and phrases are:

- *Likewise.* This word indicates that the speaker is about to show how two concepts or examples are similar.
- *On the other hand.* When you hear this phrase or something similar, you know that the speaker is about to begin discussing an opposing fact or opinion.
- *Therefore.* This word usually indicates that the speaker is about to present an effect in a cause-and-effect relationship or a logical conclusion.

- *Finally.* This word lets you know that the speaker is arriving at the end of a point or the end of the lecture.
- *To sum up.* This phrase indicates the preceding points are about to be pulled together for the main idea. Be sure to get this in your notes!

## WHAT IS MOST IMPORTANT?

Being able to separate more important information from less important information is a skill all active listeners need. Instructors often have similar ways of communicating important information. Some write key terms and concepts on the board as they lecture. Some use a PowerPoint presentation with key points bulleted. Others distribute copies of lecture outlines at the beginning of class. By picking up on these clues, you'll have an easier time determining what information your instructor considers most important.

The following behaviors also can draw your attention to important material. Your instructor may:

- pause to allow students to write down information in their notes
- repeat facts or definitions
- emphasize certain information with tone of voice
- directly tell students what information is important (e.g., "Remember this for next Tuesday's test.")
- use gestures and facial expressions to draw attention to key information
- use visual aids, such as films, television segments, life-size plastic models, and information or images on projector screens
- have students turn to certain pages in the textbook

Your instructors might not say, "This information is important." It's more likely that their behavior will give you the clues you'll need to figure out if it's important on your own. One way to pick up on these clues is to listen closely. Pay attention not only to your instructor's words but to the tone and volume of their voice as well. Another way to notice clues about important material is to observe. Even if you are listening closely to every word your instructor says, if your head is buried in your notebook the whole time, you might miss certain clues. Instead, look up from your notes from time to time to observe your instructor's actions. Hand gestures and facial expressions can indicate important information almost as clearly as words.

> If your instructor repeats something, it's probably important information to remember.

## LISAN AND LEARN

One of the benefits of active listening is that it helps you take more effective class notes. You'll learn about different note-taking methods later in this chapter. When deciding what format to use when you take notes, make sure your note-taking method encourages active listening. The LISAN method of note taking focuses on the following:

**L** *Lead instead of follow.* Think about what your instructor might say next.

**I** *Ideas.* What are the main ideas?

**S** *Signal words.* Listen for signal words that indicate transitions in the lecture. In which direction is the lecture headed?

**A** *Actively listen.* Make sure your mind stays engaged. Ask questions or make a note to yourself to seek clarification for difficult concepts later.

**N** *Notes.* Write down main ideas, key terms, and all other important information. Be selective.

## Listening Levels

Listening has to reach a certain level before it is considered active. Consider the chart to see how well you listen in class. What level are you?

| Level | Explanation |
|---|---|
| Reception | hearing words without thinking about them |
| Attention | passive listening; not making an effort to understand the information |
| Definition | entering into active listening; attaching meaning to certain facts and details but not yet organizing the material in your head |
| Integration | relating new information to your background knowledge and knowledge from previous classes |
| Interpretation | putting information into your own words; paraphrasing |
| Implication | thinking about how different pieces of information fit together; drawing conclusions |
| Application | considering how the information applies to you personally; using it in new situations |
| Evaluation | making judgments about the accuracy and relevance of the information |

Remember that active listening is a learned skill. By following the tips in this chapter, you can learn to listen at a higher level. And once you know how to apply and evaluate information as you listen, you'll be that much further on your way to becoming a successful student!

## Potential Listening Problems

With so much learning taking place by listening to the instructor speak in the classroom, a problem may occur if you can't follow the instructor well because he or she is speaking too fast or so slowly that your mind wanders. Either way, you can make the effort to gain the most from the class.

### AT BREAKNECK SPEEDS

What happens if the instructor is moving too quickly? If you're prepared for class and keeping up with your reading and still can't keep up with the lecture, you should speak up! When doing this, be specific. Avoid interrupting with a vague statement such as, "I don't understand." This kind of statement implies that you didn't prepare for class. Also, it may be frustrating to your instructor because it doesn't indicate what information you need explained more fully. Instead, show your instructor what part of the material you *did* understand by summarizing it in your own words. Then, ask a specific question. For example, you could say, "I understand that sterile technique means doing things to prevent contamination, like wearing sterile gloves and using sterile instruments. But could you explain the difference between sterile technique and aseptic technique? Are they the same?"

Occasionally, you may feel like the only student in the class who isn't keeping up. You're not alone—many students have felt this way at one point or another. If this is the case, it's probably because the other students in the class already have a greater foundation of knowledge. They may have taken prerequisite courses that you haven't. If this happens, try not to get discouraged or give up following along with the lecture. Instead, make an effort to listen more closely and continue taking notes, being careful to write down confusing terms or concepts. After class, look in your textbook or ask your instructor for clarification. This practice of writing down what you don't understand is also helpful if you meet regularly with a tutor. It gives you specific pieces of information to review.

### AT A SNAIL'S PACE

Alternatively, you may encounter instructors who present material at a much slower pace. If you allow yourself to become bored during these classes, your mind will begin to wander. To stay focused on the material, there are several tricks you can use:

- Practice summarizing information in your head. By forcing your brain to think about putting ideas into your own words, you'll stay alert.
- Try to memorize definitions of key terms as your instructor goes over them. Instead of simply reading the definitions or hearing

about them, you'll be committing them to memory for future reference.

- Predict what information your instructor will cover next. This causes you to consider how your instructor thinks. You will gain a better understanding of what your instructor expects students to know.

## When an Instructor Moves Too Slowly

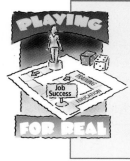

My name is Sean. I'm going to school to become a dental assistant. For the most part, I've liked my classes, but I've had to take a few boring ones, too. I had this one instructor who talked *so slowly* that I could hardly stay awake during class. Even when I brought a cup of coffee with me, I still found myself nodding off by the end of the lecture.

Then I discovered a solution. I realized it was a lot easier to stay awake if I had to think about the information and put it in my own words. So I'd just summarize in my head what my instructor was saying. It worked a lot better than caffeine!

## MAKE ADJUSTMENTS

Occasionally, you'll have to make your own adjustments for an instructor who doesn't present information clearly. In such cases, you may have to think of examples, draw conclusions, or apply new information on your own. To do these things, you'll need to maintain active listening.

Here are several tips you can use to make sure you keep listening actively:

- Remember your purpose for listening.
- Pay special attention to the beginning and end of the lecture, when your instructor might introduce and summarize key points.
- Take effective notes.
- Sit up straight to avoid feeling sleepy and to show your interest in the lecture.
- Make sure your eyes stay focused on the instructor.
- Ignore external and internal distractions by concentrating on the instructor's words.
- Analyze the material.
- Listen for main points.
- Make a note of words or concepts you don't understand so you can look them up after class.
- Adjust to the pace of the lecture.

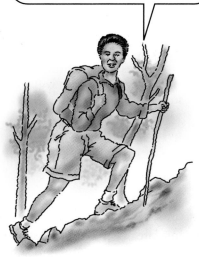

*Trying to learn new material from a poor speaker might feel like you're climbing uphill. Show that you're up for the challenge by being an active listener!*

# LEARNING IN THE CLASSROOM

So far, we've discussed how to listen actively in the classroom. But much more goes on in the classroom than just the instructor's spoken words. To be an active learner, you'll also use observational skills, your own thinking skills, note-taking skills, and much more—often all at the same time!

## Different Teaching Styles

During your time in school, you will come across many different types of instructors. One instructor may seem disorganized and another doesn't seem to cover the material in your textbook. Some instructors might not tell you exactly what you'll need to know for tests and quizzes. Although these situations may seem frustrating at first, you shouldn't use them as excuses to give up. To become a successful student, you'll need to learn to roll with the punches!

When faced with these difficult situations, use them as opportunities to engage in your own learning process. When you're an active participant, you can achieve goals other than simply learning the required material. You can accomplish things such as:

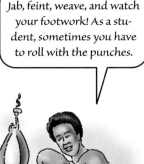

Jab, feint, weave, and watch your footwork! As a student, sometimes you have to roll with the punches.

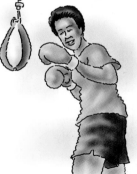

- *Improving your learning skills.* You'll use these skills not only in school but in your future career as well. Remember, learning is a lifelong process!

- *Recognizing how lecture content is organized.* Whether your instructor follows the textbook, lectures independently of the text, or uses other media should help shape your learning focus for a particular class.

- *Discovering how to measure up to your instructor's expectations.* This is also a useful skill for when you become a practicing health care professional. In the future, you may not have to answer to an instructor, but you will want to know if you're meeting your supervisor's expectations.

## Improve Your Learning Skills

Improving your learning skills also helps you succeed in the classroom. Learning skills include:

- memorization
- the ability to apply new knowledge
- interpretation of difficult material
- the ability to identify different teaching styles

It may be that an instructor is not an ineffective or bad lecturer, but one who presents material in a different way from your other instructors. Or it may be that the material in a particular class requires a different style of teaching than you're used to. When this happens, look for clues to discover your instructor's teaching style. Then use your different learning skills to help you adapt to the class.

## MEMORIZE IT!

You'll probably find that a lot of memorization is required in your introductory courses. However, your instructors may not always tell you which specific information to memorize. In these cases, look for clues to identify important information and commit it to memory.

For example, if your instructor writes a new concept or a definition on the board, you should make an effort to memorize it. Likewise, if your instructor distributes a handout depicting a diagram or a list of facts, it would be wise to remember that information as well. By learning early on to pay attention to your instructor's cues, you'll know what material to memorize before the first quiz or test.

## APPLY IT!

Some instructors focus on getting students to consider how the course material will apply to their future careers. If this is your instructor's goal, you'll do well in the course by showing that you can apply new knowledge. There are several ways in which your instructor might encourage you to do this:

- If your instructor gives many written assignments, be prepared to give examples of real-life applications in writing.
- If your instructor has students work through case studies during class, expect to see similar case studies on tests.
- If your instructor often calls students to the board to solve problems, be prepared to explain to the rest of the class how you would apply your new knowledge.

## INTERPRET IT!

In advanced science and health classes, instructors may ask students to interpret new information. This means you'll be expected to put ideas into your own words to show how well you understand the material. You'll recognize instructors who focus on interpretation by the fact that they often use class periods to ask questions and provide guidance on student responses. If your instructor uses this particular method, be sure to complete all assigned readings before class. Being prepared will allow you to participate in class discussions.

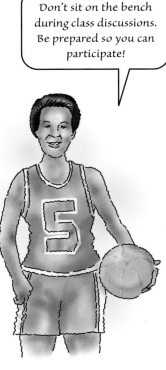

Don't sit on the bench during class discussions. Be prepared so you can participate!

## KNOW WHEN TO SHIFT GEARS

Being watchful to identify shifts in your instructor's teaching style keeps you alert and helps you follow along with the lecture. For example, the notes you take during a class discussion are different from the notes you take when your instructor gives you key terms and definitions to memorize. During a group discussion, you're focused more on ideas and the relationships between them. You won't be writing down everything said in class. In contrast, when your instructor gives you a definition to memorize, you'll need to either highlight the definition in your textbook or copy it word for word into your notes.

So, the next time your instructor interrupts a class discussion to write an important date or key term on the board, you'll identify the switch from an interpretive style of teaching to a memorization mode. You'll be able to adapt to this shift in teaching style by switching gears and recording the information from the board into your notes.

By listening actively, you'll soon become more familiar with your instructors' behavior. Pay attention to patterns in the way your instructors teach. One may tell students directly that a particular concept is important. But another may give less obvious clues, such as becoming animated or using gestures when explaining important points. Once you can recognize shifts in an instructor's teaching style, you'll begin to get more out of each lecture.

## DISCOVER HOW LECTURE CONTENT IS ORGANIZED

The content in lectures can be organized in one of two ways:

1. *Text-dependent.* In lectures where the content is text-dependent, the material is presented very similarly to how it's presented in your textbook.

2. *Text-independent.* In these lectures, instructors cite resources other than the textbook when presenting the information they consider most important.

Regardless of how closely their lectures follow the text, many instructors use media as well to help them present lecture content.

### A Textbook Case

If an instructor often conducts text-dependent lectures, it's especially important that you complete the assigned reading before class. If you're familiar with the material already, you'll have an easier time following along.

It's also important to bring your textbook to each class. As your instructor talks about sections in the text, note important ideas in the margins of your book. Highlight any passages or definitions your instructor reads aloud. If your instructor mentions that a particular section is unimportant or that you don't need to know the information it contains, cross it out.

Some students don't like to mark up their books by writing in the margins or highlighting sections of text. This is because, if you plan to sell the book back to the bookstore after the term, the bookstore will pay more for books that haven't been marked up. At first, this may sound like a good plan for the budget-conscious student. However, carefully consider whether it's really worth it. Being able to highlight and quickly refer back to important lecture points is likely well worth the few dollars difference. Actually, it's better not to sell them back at all but to keep your textbooks to build a reference library to use later on in your professional career.

## Beyond the Text

For lectures in which the content is text-independent, the focus shifts from your textbook to your notes. It's important to take effective notes during these lectures because you won't be able to refer back to your textbook for information you missed. After class, review or outline your notes to make sure you understand the key points. To gain a better understanding of the information, you may want to discuss each lecture with a classmate—you could take turns "teaching" each other the material, which will help cement it in your brain. You can also use supplementary material, such as computer software or online articles, to review concepts presented by your instructor.

Before you sit down to study any material, set study goals to remind yourself what information you need to learn. This is essential when dealing with content that doesn't appear in your textbook. You'll need to create your own learning objectives for the information in your lecture notes because the chapter objectives from your textbook may not apply.

## A Media Frenzy

A third element that affects lecture content is the use of media. Handouts, films, slide or PowerPoint presentations, plastic models, and other media give students new ways of learning material. For example, a movie might cause you to have an emotional response to a certain topic, whereas a plastic model might give you an opportunity to practice your clinical skills. With each form of media, you connect to the material in a different way. Often, this allows you to learn and understand more information than you would by simply hearing your instructor discuss it.

When dealing with media in the classroom, focus on two key questions. Ask yourself:

- Why is the instructor using this particular medium?
- How does this medium meet my learning needs?

For instance, suppose your instructor plays a television segment during class. If the segment is about a topic you've already covered, it can help you review necessary information. But if the segment introduces a new topic, it can meet your learning needs by providing you with background knowledge.

## Taking Up the Slack

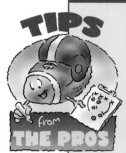

If a speaker is hard to follow, pick up the slack in the lecture by using the strategies listed in the chart.

| If your instructor doesn't . . . | You should . . . |
| --- | --- |
| explain goals for the day's lecture | set goals yourself by referring to your textbook or syllabus |
| go over information covered in the previous lecture | review your lecture notes for a few minutes before each class |
| provide an introduction or summary at the beginning and end of a lecture | write a brief summary of each lecture after class |
| supply an outline of each lecture | review the assigned reading before class or outline your notes after the day's lecture |
| give students enough time to write notes before moving on to the next topic | politely ask your instructor to repeat or clarify information |
| speak in a clear, loud tone of voice | politely ask your instructor to speak louder, or move to a closer seat, as long as you don't disrupt the class |
| answer students' questions without being sarcastic or discouraging | avoid taking your instructor's remarks personally |
| stay on topic and instead begins talking about personal experiences | think about how the instructor's stories relate to the topic |
| explain the chapter and instead reads directly from the textbook | follow along by highlighting the text your instructor reads; outline or summarize the text in your notes |
| provide the main points of the lecture | reread your textbook after class and locate main points |
| clarify confusing information or provide examples | ask your instructor to provide an example or come up with an example on your own |
| write key terms and definitions on the chalkboard | look up key terms in a dictionary or in the glossary of your textbook |

## PARTICIPATE IN CLASS

Active learning includes fully engaging with the learning process while in the classroom. Participating in class by asking the instructor questions, answering questions the instructor poses to the class, and responding to the comments of other students all help you engage more fully in the process. Be sure to try the participation techniques you learned in Chapter 4 to stay actively involved in all your classes rather than a passive student.

# Seeing Is Believing

It may seem obvious, but being able to see in the classroom is critical to your success in the course. Make sure you have a clear view of the instructor and the front of the room. Pay special attention to where visual aids, such as projector screens, are located. Be sure to choose a seat with an unobstructed view of boards and screens. The instructor may write key terms or main ideas on the board during a lecture. Being able to see this information will be helpful as you take notes.

## CHARTS AND MODELS

Instructors often use anatomical charts and plastic lifelike models, particularly in health science classes. For example, when you are learning about the human skeletal system, a full skeleton model may be used in class. Seeing the model up close will help you learn and remember the names of the bones more easily.

## SKILLS DEMONSTRATIONS

Skills demonstrations are common in many health professions classrooms. In fact, many health science classrooms are designed specifically for demonstrations and student practice sessions. It's especially important to scope out such a room and choose a seat nearest where the demonstrations are going to be given. This way, you'll be able to see everything being demonstrated.

In skills labs, students learn and practice new clinical skills, such as how to take a patient's blood pressure or count a pulse. During labs, you'll be asked to perform the skills your instructor has demonstrated. Having a clear view of in-class demonstrations will make it easier for you to learn new skills and perform them correctly.

## Getting the Most out of Class

Listening in class, watching presentations, participating in discussions and asking questions, and taking notes are key ways to increase learning in the classroom, but they're not everything. To increase your learning potential, also pay close attention to:

- information presented in handouts
- key terms or ideas the instructor writes on the chalkboard
- any questions raised by classmates and your instructor's responses to those questions
- your own opinions and thoughts about material presented by your instructor
- material that isn't covered in the textbook
- your instructor's introductory and summary statements (given at the beginning and end of each lecture)

Remember that using your personal learning style can give you an advantage in the classroom, as discussed in Chapter 5. Being aware of *how* you learn can help you increase the amount of information you understand and remember. Try to use a variety of learning techniques both to accommodate your own learning style and to increase your skills with other styles as well. Follow the tips for your own style presented in Chapter 5. Not only will you begin to perform better academically, but you'll have better communication with your instructors.

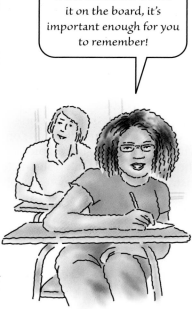

If the instructor writes it on the board, it's important enough for you to remember!

## EFFECTIVE NOTE TAKING

Another way to get the most out of your classes is to take good notes. This is a good habit to develop from the first day of class and use during the rest of the course. One of the immediate benefits of note taking is that it familiarizes you with your instructor's teaching style. Another benefit is that you are more likely to remember information after writing it down. Studies have shown that when students take notes, they remember the information included in their notes 34% of the time. Without taking notes, however, the average student remembers the same information only 5% of the time.

Note taking often involves listing main ideas and summarizing information in your own words. It keeps your brain engaged and helps you analyze information while your instructor is speaking. There are several other good reasons to take notes during lectures.

- Notes provide you with memory cues to help you review and study the information covered during class. This can be critical when the time comes to prepare for tests and quizzes.
- Lecture notes show you what material the instructor considers important. The notes can help you gauge what information will appear on tests and quizzes.
- Taking notes helps you stay more focused during the lecture. You'll more easily become familiar with and better understand new material.

This section discusses several methods all students can use to take effective notes.

## Take Notes in Class

It may seem as if some students were born with the ability to take good notes. But note taking is a learned skill! You can learn how to take effective notes by using the following tips.

- Use your own shorthand.
- Make sure your notes contain personal applications.
- Use a note-taking strategy that fits your style of learning and your instructor's style of teaching.
- Organize your notes while taking them.
- Review your notes after class, correct any unclear writing, and write a summary of the class.

### SHORTHAND HELPS YOU KEEP UP THE PACE

Develop your own shorthand for taking notes. By abbreviating words and using symbols, you'll be able to keep up with a fast-paced lecture. To improve your speed in taking notes:

- Abbreviate commonly used words. For example, the abbreviation pt. can be used for the word *patient*. You can make up your own abbreviations. Just remember to use them consistently.
- Develop shorthand symbols for other common words. For example, the symbol → means "leads to" or "causes." The symbol > means "greater than."
- Leave out conjunctions (*or, and, but*) and prepositions (*of, in, for, on, to, with*, etc.) if they aren't needed to understand the idea.
- Take a moment to think before you jot down a note. This helps you focus on one thought and write it down quickly and concisely.

- Don't try to write down the instructor's exact words except with definitions or other precise wordings.
- Don't copy text directly out of the textbook. Instead, highlight the text in your book and refer to the appropriate page number in your notes.

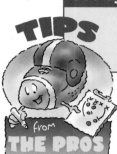

## Use Symbols + Abbr.

The chart lists some common note-taking abbreviations and symbols. Speed your note taking by using these shortcuts or coming up with your own.

> Be sure to keep a copy of your shorthand key handy when taking notes.

| Abbreviations | | Symbols | |
|---|---|---|---|
| Abt | about | ® | right |
| b/c | because | Ⓛ | left |
| Dx | diagnose or diagnosis | ↑ | increase, increased, or increasing |
| e.g. | for example | ↓ | decrease, decreased, or decreasing |
| h/a | headache | → | leads to or causes |
| Hx | history | > | more than |
| Imp | important | < | less than |
| Incl. | including | Δ | change |
| Pt | patient | ~ | about, approximately |
| Px | physical | + | and, in addition |
| Rx | treat or treatment | # | pounds or number |
| s/e | side effects | * | important or stressed by instructor |
| s/s | signs and symptoms | p̄ | after |
| w/ | with | ā | before |
| w/o | without | — | negative |
| | | c̄ | with |
| | | s̄ | without |

## APPLY IT!

Be sure to include personal applications in your notes. Write down cues to help you link new information to your previous knowledge. This not only helps you maintain active listening but will also help you study the material later.

Using someone else's lecture notes should be a last resort. Copying notes doesn't allow you to analyze the material. For this reason, borrow notes only on the rare occasions when you are unable to attend a class. You'll have an easier time learning the information if you're present for each lecture and take notes yourself.

## PEN AND PAPER ARE BETTER

Although it may seem like a wise idea, tape-recording lectures isn't the most efficient way to learn or study new material. Some of the problems with recording are:

- It increases your review/study time. It only takes a few minutes to read through your lecture notes for the day. However, listening to the entire lecture all over again takes much longer.
- A tape recording doesn't include diagrams or other important information the instructor writes on the chalkboard during a lecture.
- Even your best intentions can be thwarted by technical difficulties. Dead batteries or a poor quality recording can cause you to miss out on important information from the lecture.
- Not all instructors allow students to record their lectures. If you must use a tape recorder, ask your instructor before class.

There is one instance when tape recording might be your best option. If you ever have to miss a class, it may be helpful to have a classmate tape the lecture. In this case, listening to the lecture on tape and taking your own notes might be more beneficial than simply copying someone else's notes.

## NOTE TAKING—WHAT'S YOUR STYLE?

Develop a note-taking style that works best for you. Following are some suggestions for personalizing your method of taking notes:

- Remember how to read your own shorthand by creating a key to keep in your notebook.
- Copy down information and diagrams that your instructor writes on the chalkboard.
- Write neatly so you can use your notes when studying for quizzes and tests.
- Leave space in your notes that you can fill in later with information from your textbook.
- Read over your notes after class and make any necessary corrections.
- Separate groups of ideas by skipping a line in your notes.
- Use a color-coding system to mark groups of ideas or to emphasize important terms and concepts.

Your note-taking style also should work well with how your instructor lectures. Your notes can be formatted in several different ways. Keep your instructor's teaching style in mind when choosing the best format for your notes:

- *Outline.* This format works well with instructors who follow strict outlines and give very organized lectures.

- *Asymmetrical columns.* If your instructor frequently gives reminders ("Remember this for the test on Tuesday") or refers to your textbook during lectures ("Let's look at page 52"), this format may work best for you. See the following section "The Cornell Method of Note Taking."

- *Compare/contrast.* This format works well with an instructor who often discusses two separate topics at the same time to show how the topics are alike and different.

- *Concept map.* This format works well with instructors who provide many anecdotes or examples of a single main idea, but who don't necessarily follow a strict outline.

Another formatting tip is to leave space (2 inches or so) at the bottom of each page for a brief summary. Reviewing your notes and summarizing each page after class helps you process the information.

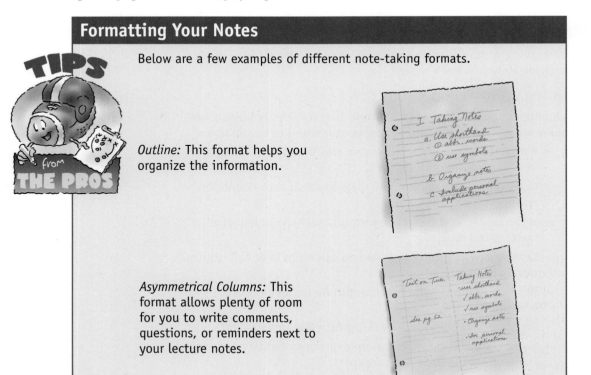

## Formatting Your Notes

Below are a few examples of different note-taking formats.

*Outline:* This format helps you organize the information.

*Asymmetrical Columns:* This format allows plenty of room for you to write comments, questions, or reminders next to your lecture notes.

*Compare/Contrast:* This format gives you an easy way of looking at how two different concepts are alike and different.

*Concept Map:* This format allows you to show how several different anecdotes or examples are connected to a single main idea.

## The Cornell Method of Note Taking

The Cornell method was developed in the 1950s at Cornell University and is still recommended by many schools because of its usefulness and flexibility. It works well for taking notes, defining priorities, and studying.

The Cornell method uses four boxes: a header, two columns, and a footer. The header is a small box across the top of the page where you write the course name, the date of the class, and other identifying information. Beneath are two columns: a narrow one on the left and a wide notes column on the right. The wide column is used for notes in an outline, list, or concepts map format. The left column is used for main ideas, key words, questions, and clarifications. Use the right column during class and the left both during the class and when reviewing your notes later. Use the box at the foot of the page to write a summary of the class. This helps you make sense of your notes during future studying. An example is shown in the illustration.

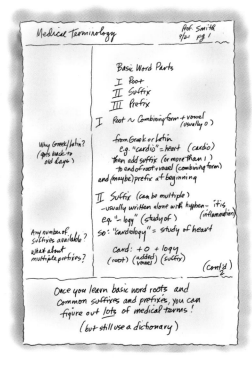

### Using Index Cards

Some students like to take notes on index cards. Cards work well also with the Cornell method. Use the lined side of the card to write your notes in class. Use one card for each key concept or topic. Use the unlined side of the card for notes normally in the left column; after class you write key words, comments, or questions here. You can then use the cards as flash cards with questions on one side and answers on the other. Write a summary of the class on a separate card and keep it on the top of the deck.

## A CINEMATIC EXPERIENCE

You may need to use a slightly different approach when taking notes on a film, television segment, or slide presentation shown during class. Although the classroom may be dark, these are not good times to tune out or doze off!

If the room is too dark for you to take notes during a film, pay close attention and jot down a brief summary or a few key points after class. If the film or TV show moves too quickly and doesn't allow you enough time to take effective notes, consider watching it again. Often, instructors place these types of presentations on reserve in the campus library. Watching the film or looking at the slides a second time will give you a chance to write down any important information you missed during class.

## FINDING A HAPPY MEDIUM

The amount of notes you take determines their effectiveness. Taking too few notes means you won't have enough material to jog your memory later. However, taking too many notes during class won't give you enough time to think about and process the information. So how do you know when enough is enough?

If your notes resemble a brief, disorganized list of facts, you're probably taking too few. In this case, focus on noting how those facts relate to one another. On the other hand, if your pen never leaves the page during class, you might be taking too many notes. Instead, work on writing down only the most important information. By finding a happy medium, your notes will become more effective.

## A Note After Class

The most important thing to remember about your notes is to review them. Try to look over your notes within 24 hours after class. It's easier to make corrections and add to your notes while the lecture is still fresh in your mind. Reviewing your notes soon after you take them also helps you commit the information to memory.

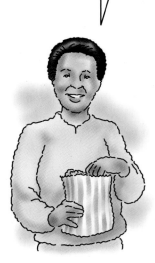

*When your instructor shows a film during class, it's not leisure time! Take notes to get the most out of it.*

**Getting Organized**

As discussed in Chapter 2, organization is critical to your success as a student. It also makes a difference in the effectiveness of your notes. Your lecture notes can be an excellent study tool, but not if they're in a disorganized jumble of papers. Take the time, either during or after class, to organize your notes. You'll thank yourself later!

# ACADEMIC READING

Do you like to read? Maybe you've been out of school for a few years but you still read newspapers, magazines, or novels? If you have been away from school for some time, it's likely that your reading has been fairly casual. The sort of concentrated reading you will do in your textbooks is very different from that casual reading. For each hour in the classroom, you may spend 2 to 3 hours studying between classes and most of that will be reading. Reading assignments are much longer than in high school and much more difficult. Textbook authors often use many technical terms and cover complex material. Some textbooks are written in a style that may be much dryer than what you're used to.

For all these reasons, it's a good idea to think about *how* to read and develop habits to remember more about what you read. Even if you don't like to read, you can develop these skills, which will pay off in a big way.

## Preparing for Class—The Need to Read

The relationship between a class of students and their instructor is comparable to the relationship between a team of athletes and their coach. Athletes must train on their own to master the basics of their sport. That way, they're prepared to refine their skills and learn about the nuances of the game when they meet with their coach. Similarly, when students work on their own to prepare for class, they become better equipped to understand and remember information from their instructor's lectures.

Even if you attend every lecture and participate in all classroom activities, you still need to prepare for class and read your course material. Reading is assigned by your instructor to help you understand concepts more fully.

Visual learners are in luck. In most courses, over 75% of the information you receive will be in the form of printed materials. This means reading is an important part of preparing for class. If you learn best by reading, here's your opportunity to take advantage of your learning strengths and put them to good use.

If you don't happen to be a visual learner, be encouraged! Regardless of your particular learning style, all students can use the same methods to develop better reading skills and improve comprehension. Ways you can get more out of reading include:

- skimming for main ideas
- using active reading techniques
- reading chapter summaries to check your comprehension

The information in the following sections will show you how to become a more successful reader. If you aren't a visual learner, you may have avoided reading in the past whenever possible. Being aware of this weakness, however, is the first step toward improving upon it. If you *are* a visual learner and you enjoy reading, the tips in this section will help you hone your preferred method of learning.

If you use these methods often enough, they'll become routine. Soon, you'll be able to read a chapter without consciously thinking about the different tasks involved in reading.

## The Anatomy and Physiology of a Textbook

First, take out one of your textbooks and give it a good looking over. Textbooks generally have a number of elements, and considering these will help prepare you for getting the most out of your reading. Here are key elements in most textbooks:

- *Preface, Introduction, Foreword.* This gives you perspective about the author's point of view. This section may also guide you on how to use the textbook and its features. It may provide hints as to why your instructor selected the book for your course.
- *Author Profile or Biography.* This helps you understand what the author considers important.
- *Table of Contents.* This is an outline of the entire book. It is very helpful in making links between the text and your course's objectives and syllabus.
- *Chapter Preview, Learning Objectives.* These sections indicate what you should pay special attention to. Compare these objectives with the course objectives stated in the syllabus.
- *Chapter Introduction.* Introductions are "must reads" because they give you a road map to the material you are about to read, directing you to notice what is truly important in the chapter or section.
- *Exercises, Activities.* These features give you a great way to confirm your understanding of the material. If you have trouble with them, you should go back and reread the section. They have the added benefit of improving your recall of the material.

- *Chapter Summary, Highlights, or Review.* It is a good idea to read this section before reading the body of the chapter. It will help you strategize about where you should invest your reading effort. Answer review questions after reading the chapter to confirm your understanding of the material.
- *Photos, Illustrations, Graphics.* Many students are tempted to skip over graphic material. Don't! Take the time to read and understand all graphics. They increase your understanding and, because they engage different learning styles, they create different memory links to help you remember the material. Use your critical thinking skills to understand why each illustration is present and what it means.

Paying attention to these textbook elements before you begin a reading assignment helps set you up for a successful experience. Now you can begin the actual reading process.

## The Steps of Effective Reading

With a newspaper or magazine, you probably just start reading from the top. Maybe you look over at a photo or illustration first, but generally you just read from the start to the end. You could do it this way with a textbook too, but you'd not learn nearly as well as you can using a more structured approach. Try using the following steps.

### START BY SKIMMING

Before you begin reading a chapter, flip though the pages and skim the material first. Doing this will give you a chance to look at the general organization of the chapter and identify key points. The purpose of skimming is to get your brain in gear so you'll absorb more information during active reading. By taking the time to skim over the chapter first, you'll give your brain the time it needs to begin organizing information in your head. This means you'll be able to mentally file information as soon as you begin reading. Not only does skimming allow you to understand the material more quickly, it also helps you to remember more of what you read.

When skimming a chapter, follow these guidelines:

1. Look at the illustrations, graphs, charts, and tables. Read any captions.
2. Read the chapter introduction (usually located in the first paragraph).
3. Read the section headings throughout the chapter.
4. Take note of emphasized words in bold or italics as you flip through the pages.
5. Read the chapter summary (usually located in the closing paragraph).

Graphic elements, such as charts and tables, illustrate important concepts covered in the chapter. Often, graphics provide snapshot views of the same information it may take several pages of text to explain. If you glance at each graphic element while skimming a chapter, you'll give yourself a quick preview of the material.

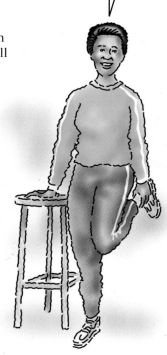

> Skimming a chapter before reading it is like stretching your muscles before running a race. You need to make sure your brain is prepared to learn new information!

### Build a Solid Foundation

When preparing to read a difficult chapter, make sure you first have some background knowledge of the topics covered. When you have a good foundation of knowledge on which to build, you'll have an easier time understanding complex new ideas.

For example, suppose a dental assistant and an experienced radiology technician both read a section in a textbook on using contrast media in certain x-ray procedures. Which individual would be able to comprehend the material more quickly and easily? Although both people may have had some experience taking x-rays, the radiology technician is likely to have a better foundation of knowledge in this particular area. The technician's background and experience would give him or her an advantage over the dental assistant, who has not had the opportunity of working with contrast media. Even the technician's familiarity with the vocabulary used to describe such procedures would make it easier for him or her to read and understand the text.

As a student, how can you expand your foundation of knowledge? One way to give yourself some background information is to read an online or magazine article on the topic. Another way to prepare for reading a difficult chapter is to attend a lecture or seminar on a related topic. At the very least, you'd become familiar with the vocabulary used in the chapter. By the time you sat down to read your textbook, you would be able to focus your energy on trying to understand the concepts presented, rather than having to try to figure out what specific words mean.

### Take a Look at the Structure

Another tactic to use when skimming text is looking at how the chapter is organized. The chapter may be structured in several different ways:

- *Subject development or definition structure.* These paragraphs present a single concept and then list supporting details. Introductory paragraphs usually are structured this way.
- *Sequence structure.* These paragraphs usually include signal words, such as *first, second, next, then,* and *finally.* The information in these paragraphs is presented in sequential order. Numbered lists also fall into this category.

- *Compare and contrast structure.* These paragraphs discuss how two or more concepts are alike and different. Words that signal comparisons include *both, similarly, too,* and *also.* Contrasting statements may include the signal words *yet, but, however,* or *on the other hand.*
- *Cause-and-effect structure.* These paragraphs often include signal words or phrases, such as *cause, effect, due to, in order to, resulting from,* and *therefore.* These paragraphs explain how one idea or event results from another idea or event.

Once you identify how the chapter is organized, you'll be on your way to pinpointing the most important information. This will help you focus when the time comes to read the full chapter.

## READY, SET, READ!

After you've skimmed the chapter, you can begin reading actively. But note that active reading goes beyond simply recognizing the words on each page. It includes using other tactics to aid your comprehension. In order to make sure you're reading actively, try putting some of the following tips into practice.

- Read aloud.
- Take notes or draw graphics as you read. (The Cornell note-taking method works well for reading also.)
- Write down any questions you have about confusing concepts or ideas.
- Think about how information in the chapter relates to important points outlined in the table of contents (or outlined at the beginning of the chapter).
- Make a note of any difficult sections you'd like to read a second time.

### Stay Focused

Active reading requires concentration. Here are some basic guidelines to help you stay focused. (Chapter 8 provides additional study tips.)

- Read during the time of day you are most alert.
- Avoid trying to read too much at one time. When you start to feel your mind wandering, take a 5-minute break.
- Find a quiet place to read. Avoid distractions, such as watching TV or listening to loud music.
- Sit in a comfortable (but not too comfortable!) chair in order to stay awake and alert while reading.
- Supply yourself with a healthy snack and water to avoid getting distracted by being hungry or thirsty.

Help yourself avoid distractions by finding a quiet place to read.

## Postgame Highlights

As you actively read each chapter, highlight important ideas or mark them with sticky notes. You can also make notes right in the margins. Just be careful not to mark too much text. If 90% of the material on every page is highlighted, it doesn't truly show which ideas are most important. But a chapter that is highlighted correctly is an excellent study tool. Being able to locate key ideas quickly will help you study more efficiently.

When deciding which text to highlight, think about what should be considered truly "important" material. Here are some hints:

- Highlight any information your instructor emphasizes in class. If your instructor considers a particular topic important, chances are that topic may appear on a test or quiz.
- Highlight portions of text that answer any questions you came up with while skimming the chapter.
- Look for and highlight topic sentences. These sentences generally include the main idea(s) in each paragraph.

Highlighting can help you find important information later, but keep in mind that it doesn't actually help you learn the material. To learn the information, spend a few extra minutes summarizing the text you highlighted in your own words. If you prefer, create a chart or diagram instead to illustrate key points. This helps you process the information and commit it to memory.

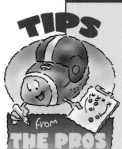

## Bright Idea: Highlighting Text

By highlighting text and making notes in the margins of your textbook, you'll remember more of what you read. You'll also be able to locate key ideas later when studying for the next test or quiz. Keep these tips in mind as you read.

- Read the entire paragraph or section before highlighting any of it.
- Highlight portions of text that answer any questions you thought of while skimming the chapter.
- Look for items presented in sequential order and number them accordingly.
- Highlight key terms, names, dates, and places.
- Summarize main ideas in the margins.
- Insert a question mark next to confusing paragraphs or sentences. Write any questions or comments you may have in the margins.
- Mark any information your instructor considers important with a star or exclamation point.
- Highlight important information in the table of contents or create a list of the most important topics.

## Make It Personal

Another way to make sure you're reading actively is to connect with the material on a personal level. By making the information more personal, you'll have an easier time remembering it. You can do this by:

- *Making associations.* For example, you might be able to remember an important date by associating it with the birthday of someone you know. (Chapter 8 discusses associations in more detail.)
- *Having an emotional response to the material.* Reacting to the information you read will make it more memorable.
- *Drawing pictures to illustrate different concepts.* A picture might be easier to remember than a paragraph of text.

## Know the Lingo

Reading actively also involves making sure you understand the vocabulary used to describe new concepts. You should always determine the meaning of an unfamiliar word before continuing your reading. In scientific texts especially, it's important to know the meaning of the technical terms used. Knowing the vocabulary makes your job of understanding the material much easier. For example, suppose you are reading a passage discussing what happens to the body during a myocardial infarction. Knowing that *myocardial infarction* is the medical term for "heart attack" would help you understand the passage more readily.

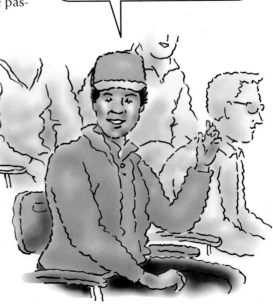

A baseball game makes a lot more sense if you're familiar with the lingo. The same is true for reading scientific texts. If you don't know a word, look it up!

When you notice an unfamiliar word, first try to figure out its meaning from context clues. Context clues can include other words or sentences that provide hints about the word's meaning. They also can include root words, prefixes, and suffixes. If you're unable to determine the word's meaning from the context, look it up in a dictionary or glossary. Saying it aloud will help you remember it. Then make a note of the definition and pronunciation in the margin of your textbook or in your notes. If the word appears once in the chapter, it may appear again.

When skimming a chapter, you may notice many unfamiliar words. It may be helpful to look up all the definitions before you begin actively reading the text.

*Read Chapter Summaries*

In most textbooks, all chapters are formatted similarly. The chapter summary usually appears toward the end of the chapter in the form of a summary paragraph, bulleted statements, or review questions.

One of the last steps in active reading is reviewing the chapter summary. Read the chapter summary and refer back to the table of contents to make sure you understood the key points of the chapter. If there are sections you didn't understand, reread them or make a note to ask your instructor for clarification.

When rereading, try using a different method from what you used during your first active reading of the chapter. You can adjust the speed of your reading by reading a particular section more slowly, for example. Reading aloud is another method. When rereading text, make an effort to understand each sentence before continuing. Think about how each new concept you encounter relates to other information in the chapter.

## Game Plan for Reading

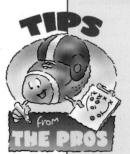

- *Pace yourself.* Unless it is very short, divide the assignment into smaller blocks rather than trying to read it all at once. If you have a week to do the assignment, for example, divide the work into five daily blocks, leaving an extra day for review.
- *Schedule your reading.* Try to read at the time of day when you are most alert.
- *Choose the right space.* Read in a quiet, well-lit space. Sit in a comfortable chair with good support. The library is an excellent option. Don't read in bed because that space is associated with sleeping.
- *Avoid distractions.* Active reading takes place in short-term memory. With every distraction, you lose continuity and have to restart. Multitasking—listening to music or texting while you read—makes for poor reading comprehension and makes the reading take much longer.
- *Prevent reading fatigue.* Give yourself a 5- to 10-minute break every hour. Put down the book, walk around, have a healthy snack, stretch, or do deep knee bends. You'll feel refreshed and be better able to stay focused.
- *Read more difficult assignments early* in your scheduled reading time when you are freshest.
- *Stay interested.* Actively go looking for answers that pop up in your mind as you read. Carry on a mental conversation with the author.

## Use Your Reading Notes Before Class

Review your textbook and create a note-taking outline before each lecture. This familiarizes you with the material and helps to organize your notes. By locating key terms and main ideas beforehand, you'll provide yourself with a basic outline to follow and fill in during the lecture. In essence, your note-taking outline is your "road map" for the lecture. By using it, there's less chance of getting lost!

To determine which terms and concepts to include in your outline, follow these steps:

1. Look at the general layout of the chapter. Make a mental note of each section's length—longer sections will need more space in your outline.

2. Read the introductory paragraph. The first paragraph in a chapter often lists main ideas.

3. Review any graphs, charts, or diagrams.

4. Search for any bold or italic words. If a word or phrase is emphasized in the chapter, it should be included in your outline.

5. Look over passages you highlighted while reading, including margin notes, questions, and other notes.

6. Read the closing paragraph. The last paragraph in a chapter usually summarizes important information and draws conclusions.

*Taking notes without a basic outline is like driving without directions. It's easy to get lost!*

During the lecture, fill in any gaps left in your outline. Add to it by including information from the lecture that is not provided by your textbook.

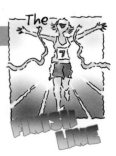

## CHAPTER SUMMARY

- Develop your active listening skills to get the most out of every class.
- Avoid behaviors that can interfere with active listening.
- When listening actively, identify main ideas and pay attention to signal words.
- Use techniques to compensate for different lecture styles and become an active participant in your own learning process.
- Learning involves several skills, including memorizing, applying, and interpreting new information.

- Develop a note-taking style that works for you. Keep your instructor's lecturing style in mind when deciding how to format your notes.
- Reading is a multipart process that includes skimming, active reading, and later reviewing and rereading.
- Give yourself a road map to follow during class by creating a note-taking outline.

## REVIEW QUESTIONS

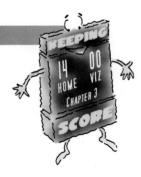

1. List at least five behaviors that could be interfering with your ability to listen actively in class.
2. How would you cope with an instructor who moves too slowly?
3. Which note-taking format would work best in a class where the instructor routinely gives a lot of anecdotes and examples to illustrate a single main idea?
4. What should you do with your class notes after you've written them in class?
5. What are at least three things you can do to make sure you're reading actively?

## CHAPTER ACTIVITIES

1. Group Exercise: Using a highlighter, read the first five pages of this chapter and highlight important passages following the guidelines given in this chapter. Then go back through these pages, looking only at what you have highlighted, and mark with a large penciled asterisk one key concept that would most likely be on a quiz covering this chapter. Finally, get together in groups of three or four students and compare what you have highlighted and marked with the asterisk. Talk about how you know what is most important here.
2. Analysis Exercise: Select a few pages of notes you took in one class session of a different course at any time *before* reading this chapter. Examine these notes to see how well they follow the guidelines suggested in the "Take Notes in Class" section of this chapter. What could you have done differently to improve the process of taking notes in class and the resulting notes?

# Communication Skills

***On completion of this chapter and the learning activities you will be able to:***

- Know why it's important for health care professionals to have good communication skills

- Be comfortable speaking informally in class and in formal presentations

- Describe the structural parts of an academic writing assignment

- Successfully use the steps of the writing process

- Effectively research information using the library and the Internet

- Participate with others in group projects

- Communicate successfully via a computer

To succeed as a student, you'll need to learn how to express yourself both through speaking and writing. This involves developing and using good communication skills both as a student and in your future career as a health professional. In this chapter, we'll discuss how to enhance your learning by speaking out in class and giving successful class presentations, whether individually or as part of a group project. You'll also learn about academic writing and how to use the writing process to ensure you do your best. Finally, we'll examine the role of computers in communication, from best email practices to online courses. All these topics involve core principles of communication. Effective communication skills are essential in all health careers. Develop yours now as a student and you'll thank yourself in the future!

# SPEAKING

During your time as a student, you may be required to give a few speeches or oral presentations. Much of your speaking in public, however, will be more informal. Whether you're asking a question during a lecture or participating in a group discussion, you should use good public speaking skills. When you're able to express yourself, you'll receive better answers to your questions and you'll also get more out of group discussions.

> I used to be so afraid to speak in front of others! Now, I'm over it.

## Me? Speak in Public?

If speaking to a group of people makes you feel nervous, nauseous, or as if you'd rather stay in bed and avoid the situation altogether, know that you're not alone. *Glossophobia*, the fear of public speaking, is considered by some to be the most common phobia.

Researchers aren't sure exactly what causes this fear. However, most agree that having a bad or embarrassing experience with public speaking is usually a major contributor. There's nothing like the embarrassment of getting up in front of a group of people and stumbling over your words (or forgetting them altogether) to make you want to avoid doing so ever again. Fortunately, there are tips you can use to improve your ability to speak up in a group setting.

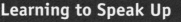

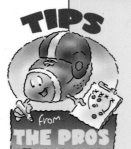

### Learning to Speak Up

Follow this step-by-step process to relax yourself before speaking up in class.

- Acknowledge your fear and admit to yourself that you're nervous about public speaking. It's very difficult to overcome a fear that "doesn't exist." Remember that stage fright is completely normal.

- Understand that your instructor and other students are not looking for faults. They likely don't even know that you're nervous and won't see your anxiety.

- Reassure yourself that you have something important to say and that your instructor and your classmates are interested in hearing it.

- Think about what you are going to say. This will give you a chance to calm your nerves. When you speak, stay focused on *what* you're saying, not *how* others are viewing you.

- Be confident. This will command everyone's interest. It may help you feel self-assured if you jot your question or comment in your notes before raising your hand to speak.

- Speak loudly and clearly. If everyone hears you the first time, you will avoid having to repeat yourself.

# Speaking Informally in Class

As mentioned previously, most of your "public" speaking will occur informally when you speak in the classroom. You might be asking a question, answering a question, or giving your perspective about someone else's comment. We call this informal speaking because the situation does not involve planning ahead to deliver a more formal presentation—a situation we'll look at later in this chapter.

Even though participating in class discussions is less formal, it still helps to be prepared and follow some basic guidelines. Start with the general principles for class participation described in Chapter 4.

### FIRST, ORGANIZE YOUR THOUGHTS

The first thing to remember is to organize your thoughts. Make sure you have read assigned material before class so that you have good background information for the lecture. During the lecture, pay attention and listen closely to make sure your instructor hasn't already addressed the question you're about to ask. Then, ask directly. There is no need to beat around the bush. Go ahead and ask for clarification of an idea or challenge a statement that seems contradictory. In most classrooms, students are encouraged to participate in this way.

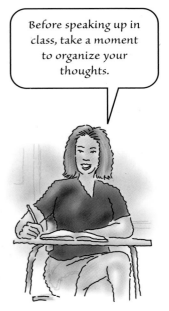

*Before speaking up in class, take a moment to organize your thoughts.*

Don't ever feel your question is "stupid." If you have paid attention in class and did assigned reading but you still don't understand something, you have every right to ask. Many other students in the class are probably wondering the same thing—and they'll be happy you took the initiative to ask!

### COME TO THE POINT

As described in Chapter 4, there's a right way and a wrong way to go about seeking clarification during a lecture. First, choose carefully your moment to speak. How the instructor moves and gestures, and the looks on his or her face, not only adds meaning to the words but also cues you when it's a good time to ask a question or stay silent.

Then think about what you will say. The wrong way is to interrupt class with a vague statement such as, "I don't get it." Instead, it's better to state briefly and in your own words what you *do* understand and then ask your question.

For example, suppose your radiology instructor is explaining how to position patients for different types of x-rays. If you need clarification, you could say, "I understand that in both the recumbent and supine positions, the patient should be lying down. But what is the difference between the two positions?" This statement clearly shows that you understand at least part of the information. It's an effective question because it comes to the point and tells your instructor exactly which part of the material you don't understand.

On the other hand, suppose you encounter a situation where you want to challenge a statement that seems to contradict your background knowledge of a particular topic. Let's say your class is having a discussion about patient privacy rights. Your instructor says, "State law requires that if a patient is diagnosed with a sexually transmitted disease, that information must be reported to the local health department." In a previous course, however, you learned that a patient's diagnosis is confidential. Your instructor's statement seems to contradict what you've already learned about patient confidentiality. How would you form a respectful question to challenge your instructor's statement?

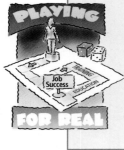

## Speaking Up

Hi, my name is Suki. I'm studying to become a lab technician. In one of the first courses I took, it was really hard to keep up with the instructor. But I was afraid to ask questions in front of everyone else in class. The few times I tried, I was so nervous that I raised my hand and then completely forgot what I was going to say.

But then I started writing down my questions so I could read them after the instructor called on me. It was so much easier! Writing down what I wanted to say gave me the time I needed to organize my thoughts. It also kept me from being too nervous and having my mind go blank.

## PARTICIPATE—GROUP DISCUSSIONS

A good way to practice speaking up in class is to participate in group discussions with your classmates. These situations provide you with low-stress opportunities to express your thoughts and ask questions. Once you become comfortable with speaking to a group of your peers, you'll gain confidence to speak up in other situations, such as asking your instructor for clarification.

Once you are comfortable speaking in class, be sure not to overdo it or dominate a discussion. Be sensitive to the needs of other students and give them the chance to ask their questions, too.

## For Future Use

The speaking skills you develop as a student will be useful throughout your career. You can bet that at some point, a situation will arise where you need to clarify a physician's instructions. You'll be thankful for all the practice you had in class communicating with your instructors! As a health care professional, you can apply the same principles you used in class when asking your supervisors for clarification.

1. First, organize your thoughts in order to ask a direct question.
2. Then, come to the point while remembering to be respectful and to use your critical thinking skills.

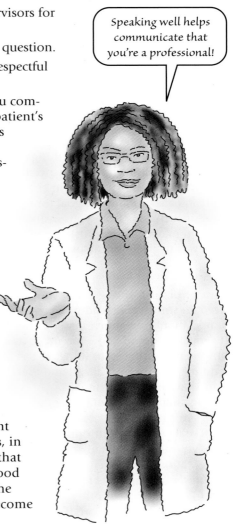

*Speaking well helps communicate that you're a professional!*

You'll also need to have good speaking skills when you communicate with patients. For example, when gathering a patient's medical history, you'll be required to ask direct questions and clarify the patient's responses. In this case, you'll need to be able to form clear, easily understandable questions to obtain the information you need. It also will be important to make sure you understand the patient's responses correctly before recording the information in a medical chart.

Good speaking skills, and good communication skills in general, are very important in the health care professions. Eventually, you'll be required to use your skills on a daily basis. Just remember that the best way to develop good skills is to practice!

## Giving Presentations

A formal presentation, another form of public speaking, involves preparation outside of class and sometimes significant research and planning. That part of the process is actually similar to writing a paper for a class or even studying for an exam. What's different is this preparation leads to a presentation given in class, in front of other students and the instructor—a situation that usually makes students *very* nervous. But relax—with good planning and communication skills, you can develop the ability to give good presentations and you may even become a classroom star!

Begin by making sure you understand the exact requirements of the assignment. What's the topic and how long should it be? Then you can begin planning. Class presentations are not difficult if you follow these six basic steps:

1. Analyze your audience and goals.
2. Plan, research, and organize your content.
3. Draft and revise the presentation.
4. Prepare visual aids.
5. Practice the presentation.
6. Deliver the presentation.

## WHO'S YOUR AUDIENCE? WHAT'S YOUR POINT?

In most class presentations, the first question seems obvious: other students and the instructor. Check the assignment, however—maybe you're supposed to address the class as if they were patients in a health care setting? Even if the audience is your class, you still need to think about what they already know and don't know about your topic. How much background information do they already have based on previous lectures and reading? Be careful not to give a boring recap of things they already know. But it may be important to show how your specific topic fits in with subjects that have been discussed already in class.

Think also about your goal for the presentation. The assignment instructions from your instructor may provide the goal, but you may need to adjust it to what you can cover well in the time you're given for the presentation.

> In a presentation, it's better to cover a smaller topic well and meet your goal than to try too much with a larger topic and not cover it fully.

## PLAN, PLAN, PLAN

Start by brainstorming about your topic. You may also need do some more reading or research. Don't worry at first about how much material you're gathering. It's much better to know too much and then pick out the most important things to say in your allotted time than to rush ahead and then realize you don't have enough material.

Organizing a presentation or speech is similar to organizing topics in a paper for class (see *Structurally Speaking* in the Writing for Classes section). Introduce your topic and state your main idea, go into more detail about specific ideas in the body of the presentation, and conclude. Look for a logical order for the body of the presentation. Some topics might be covered in a chronological (time) order, whereas others are best developed through a compare-and-contrast organization. If your goal is to persuade, sort out your separate arguments and build to the strongest or most important. Put similar ideas together and think about how you'll need to transition between very different ideas.

While researching your topic and outlining your main points, also start thinking about visual aids for the presentation.

## DRAFT AND REVISE

You don't need to actually write out the presentation in full sentences and paragraphs because you shouldn't read it aloud—that makes for a dull presentation. Some students speak well from brief phrases written on note cards, whereas others prefer a more detailed outline.

You can't know for sure how long your presentation will last until you rehearse it, but try to estimate the time while drafting it. Figure that it takes 2 to 3 minutes to speak the amount of writing on a standard double-spaced page—but with visual aids, pauses, and audience interaction, it may take longer. This is only a rough guide, but you might start out thinking of a 10-minute presentation as the equivalent of a 3- to 4-page paper.

As you draft your speaking notes, consider questions like these:

- Am I going on too long about minor points?
- Do I have good explanations and reasons for my main points? Do I need more data or better examples? Where would visual aids be most effective?
- Am I using the best words for this topic and this audience? Should I be more or less informal in the way I talk about my topic?
- Does it all hold together and flow well from one point to the next? Do I need a transition when I shift from one idea to another?

## PREPARE VISUAL AIDS

Most presentations gain from visuals and, with visual technology used in many classrooms, visual aids are often expected. Consider all possibilities when choosing appropriate visuals:

- charts, graphs
- maps
- photos, other images
- video clips
- handouts (only when necessary—otherwise may be distracting)

## PRACTICE, PRACTICE, PRACTICE

Practice is the most important step in preparing. It also helps you get over stage fright and gain the confidence that you'll do a good job.

Practice first alone, either to a mirror or in an empty room where you imagine people sitting (so that you can move your eyes around the room to this "audience"). Do not read your notes aloud but speak in sentences natural for you. Glance down at your notes only briefly, then look up immediately to the mirror or around the room. Time yourself but don't obsess about using precisely the exact number of minutes your instructor requested. If your presentation is way off, however, adjust your outlined notes.

Once you feel good about delivering your content from your notes, practice some more to work on your delivery. You might want to record or videotape your presentation or ask a friend or roommate to watch your presentation.

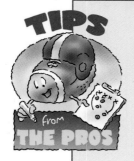

## Using Visual Aids

Use the available technology, whether an overhead projector or PowerPoint screen, or a flip chart or posters. Always check the assignment to confirm your instructor's expectations for your use of visual aids. You might also talk to your instructor about resources and software for designing your visuals. Follow these guidelines:

- Design your visuals carefully. Use a simple, neutral background. Minimize the amount of text in visuals. Don't simply present word outlines of what you are saying.

- Don't use more than two pictures in a slide and use two only to make a direct comparison. Image montages are hard to focus on and distracting.

- Don't put a table of numbers in a visual aid. If you need to illustrate numerical data, use a graph. Don't use too many visuals or move through them so quickly that the audience gives all its attention to them rather than to you.

- Practice your presentation using your visual aids, because they will affect your timing.

- Explain visuals when needed but not when they're obvious.

- Keep your eyes on your audience, only briefly glancing at visuals to stay in synch with them.

---

- Practice a good opening to capture the audience's attention. Start with a striking fact or example (illustrating an issue, a problem), a brief interesting or humorous anecdote (historical, personal, current event), a question to the audience, or an interesting quotation. Then relate the opening to your topic and your main point and move into the body of the presentation.

- Try to speak in your natural voice, not a monotone as if you were just reading aloud.

- Practice making changes in your delivery speed and intensity to emphasize key points in your presentation.

- Don't keep looking at your notes. It's fine if you use words that are different from those you wrote down—the more you rehearse without looking at your notes, the more natural you will sound.

- Be sure you can pronounce all new words and technical terms correctly. Practice saying them slowly and clearly to yourself until you can say them naturally.

- Don't forget transitions. A reader notices it when a writer moves on to a new point (with a heading in the text, a paragraph break, or a transitional phrase), and listeners also need a cue that you're moving to a new idea. Practice phrases such as "Another important reason for this is . . ." or "Now let's move on to why this is so. . . ."

- Watch out for all those little "filler" words people so often use in conversation, such as *like, you know, well*, and *uh*.

- Pay attention to your body language when practicing. Stand up straight and tall in every practice session so that you become used to it. Unless you have to use a fixed microphone in your presentation, practice moving around while you speak. Make natural gestures. Keep your eyes moving and making eye contact with the audience when you present. Practice smiling and occasionally pausing at key points.

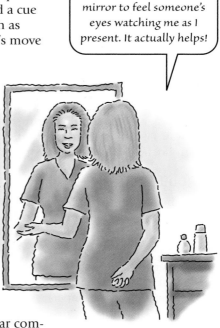

I practice in front of a mirror to feel someone's eyes watching me as I present. It actually helps!

## DELIVER THE PRESENTATION

On presentation day, get plenty of sleep and eat a healthy breakfast. Don't drink too many caffeinated drinks because that may make you hyper and nervous. Wear comfortable shoes and appropriate professional clothing that won't restrict you or make you self-conscious as you move around before the audience.

Remember: the audience is on your side! If you're still nervous before your presentation, take a few deep breaths. Rehearse your opening lines in your mind so that you don't have to look at your notes immediately when starting. Instead, look out and around your audience. Smile as you move to the front of the room. You'll see some friendly faces smiling back encouragingly.

# WRITING FOR CLASSES

Writing, like speaking, is an important communication skill. As a student, you'll most likely be required to write essays, reports, and research papers. The writing skills you develop in school will carry over into your professional career as well. As an allied health professional, you'll need solid writing skills for recording accurate and concise information in patient charts and medical records.

Writing skills can be helpful for a number of other reasons, one of which is securing your first job. A well-written résumé and cover letter can help you get your foot in the door and get an interview, as discussed in Chapter 12. Even in email messages, being able to express yourself well shows that you are intelligent and competent. It also effectively gets your message across to the person with whom you are communicating. Good writing skills help you avoid misunderstandings that can result from poor communication.

## Structurally Speaking

Whether you're writing a 15-page paper or a brief essay, your writing assignments should be structured in roughly the same way. Like an oral presentation, formal writing includes an introduction, a body, and a conclusion.

> Spice up your introduction by beginning with a brief story, asking a question, or presenting an interesting fact.

### INTRODUCTION

Always begin your written assignments with an introduction. The introduction should interest the reader in the topic you're about to discuss. Your introduction can be structured in a number of different ways. It can:

- be centered on a thesis statement (a thesis statement is a statement of the opinion or idea to be discussed in your paper)
- present a problem or ask a question that you intend to answer
- describe a dramatic event or incident
- provide interesting statistics
- set a scene
- relate a short story

For example, in a persuasive essay, your introduction could begin by presenting a topic. Then, your thesis statement could include the main point you intend to prove about that topic.

Keep in mind that your introduction doesn't have to be the first thing you write. Even if you start with a basic outline and have a general idea of how you'd like to approach your topic, it's easy to get stuck on the introduction. If this happens, try working on other portions of the paper for a while and come back to it. Your introduction will be easier to write once you have a clear purpose in mind.

The introduction should be roughly 5% to 15% of the length of your entire paper. It needs to be informative but to the point. It should be interesting without giving away too much detail. For these reasons, it takes time and effort to write a good introduction. You may want to revise it again after you've completed your paper.

## BODY

You do most of your writing in the body, which makes up about 70% to 90% of a paper's total length. The body of a paper presents details that support your thesis. This may include:

- background information about your topic
- facts and supporting research
- explanations of key terms or phrases used throughout the paper
- quotes from other credible sources
- different arguments against your thesis and your responses to those arguments

## CONCLUSION

A strong conclusion ends the discussion presented in the paper and makes the reader think. To accomplish this, the conclusion needs to do more than blandly summarize main points. To write a strong conclusion, consider including:

- a quotation that relates to or sums up your thesis
- a question for the reader to consider
- encouragement for the reader to act in support of your idea
- one last example or story to reiterate your point

## BIBLIOGRAPHY AND REFERENCES

The bibliography is a list of the sources you used to write your paper. It's important because it helps you back up the information included in your paper and gives credit to your sources of research. Whether you gathered information from a book, a website, a television program, or a magazine article, each source must be included in your bibliography. A bibliography only shows the general sources, however. For quotations, specific statistics, and the theories and opinions of others, you'll need to include specific references, either as footnotes or numbered endnotes. Your instructor will tell you the specific reference format to use.

## APPENDIX

You probably won't need to include an appendix with each formal writing assignment you complete. An appendix is only necessary when you need to include other supportive materials that do not belong or cannot fit in the body of your paper. A few examples of such materials are:

- a list of key terms and definitions
- photos, illustrations, or figures
- tables, charts, maps, and other graphic elements

# The Writing Process

So you've decided on the type of paper you're going to write. You know it needs to have an introduction, a body, and a conclusion. What next? First, carefully reread the assignment to make sure you fully understand it. Is your topic appropriate? Are you expected to do research? How long should the final result be? When you are clear about all aspects of the assignment, you're ready to start the process.

Writing a paper involves several steps in a process. The writing process is a time-tested method to ensure you do your best on the paper.

1. Set your schedule.
2. Select a topic.
3. Collect information.
4. Organize the information.
5. Evaluate the information.
6. Create an outline.
7. Write a first draft.
8. Revise the first draft.
9. Finalize the paper.

## SCHEDULING

A good way to set up a schedule for writing a paper is to work backward from the due date listed in your syllabus. Then, mark the following on your calendar and weekly planner:

- due date for the paper
- amount of time you need to revise the paper
- amount of time you need to write the first draft
- date you should complete your research
- date you need to begin research

When scheduling your time, be generous! Unexpected problems can arise, making some steps take longer than you anticipated. For example, you may go to the library to find that a book you need has already been checked out. Or you may find that you need extra time to evaluate and organize the materials you gathered. Whatever delays may occur, you can avoid stress by building in extra time for the full process.

Another aspect that may affect your writing schedule is the paper's length. Sometimes it's hard to predict how much work you'll need to do to complete the assignment. When considering how much time to allow yourself to write the paper, keep the following in mind:

- the required length of the paper
- the amount of time you have before the due date
- the amount of research you're expected to do
- the number of references your instructor requires you to have

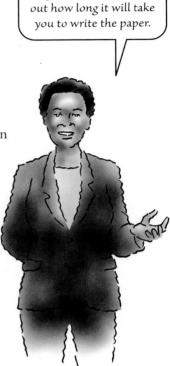

Use the required page length to help you figure out how long it will take you to write the paper.

## SELECTING A TOPIC

If your instructor assigns a specific topic, you won't have to worry about this stage of the writing process. If not, your instructor may give you a list of acceptable topics or guidelines for creating your own topic. When thinking about possible topics, select one that captures your interest. When you write about a subject that interests you, you'll be better motivated to work on the paper. Also, be sure to select a topic that you'll be able to research adequately. You'll have a hard time completing an assignment that requires a lot of research on an obscure topic.

Good places to search for topic ideas include:

- the table of contents in your textbook
- your lecture notes
- brainstorming sessions with your study group
- magazines, journals
- websites

Just remember to keep your topic fairly narrow. A more focused topic means a more focused writing process and a better paper. When looking for a topic, try to find a balance. Your topic should provide you with enough material to complete the assignment, but it should be focused enough so that you can explain it fully in your paper.

One way to see if a topic is well defined or focused enough is to think about your thesis statement and the title of the paper. A good title is clear and appealing. The reader should know what the paper is about just by reading the title. However, if you come up with a title before writing the paper, keep in mind that the title isn't permanent and may need to be changed after the paper has been completed. Sometimes, it's simply a good exercise to think about the main point you'd like to communicate in your paper. Doing so may help you decide on a particular topic.

## COLLECTING INFORMATION

When gathering information for your paper, it's probably wise to begin at the library. Start by looking up your topic in the library's computer system or reference books for the subject. (See the later section *Library Research*.)

## Other Sources of Information

In addition to the library, other excellent sources of information include:

- *Interviews with professors or experts in the field.* Conducting interviews will prepare you for future clinical work, when you may have to conduct information-gathering interviews with patients. In both cases, the process is similar.

  1. Be prepared. Make a list of the questions you'd like to ask. Make sure the most important questions are at the top of your list.

  2. During the interview, keep the conversation focused. If you only have a limited amount of time, try to avoid talking about things unrelated to your questions.

  3. Finally, when gathering information for a paper, you may wish to audiotape the interview in addition to taking notes. This can help you remember quotes accurately. It also gives you a way to review any information you may have missed. Just remember to ask permission first. You can do this when scheduling the interview to avoid putting your interviewee on the spot when you meet; not everyone is comfortable with being recorded.

- *Surveys and statistics.* The results of professional surveys may add to the information for your paper. But you can conduct your own surveys as well. Statistics can be calculated after you receive responses to your survey. For example, suppose you surveyed 50 subjects and 15 of those individuals answered *yes* to a particular question. The other 35 subjects answered *no.* Your statistics for that question would be 30% answering *yes* and 70% answering *no.* These results could then be used in your paper to support or argue against a particular point.

- *Resources on the Internet.* When searching for information online, there are two very important guidelines to keep in mind.

  1. Make sure the material you find is reliable. (See the *Websites* section later in this chapter.)

  2. Remember to cite any online information you use in your paper. Your instructor will be able to tell you which reference format to use when citing information. You'll most likely need to include the Web address, site owner, date the site was last updated (if available), and the date you accessed the information.

- *Unbiased observations.* Your own unbiased observations can be used as a source of information for your paper. However, the key word here is *unbiased.* There are several methods you can use to avoid allowing your own opinions to cloud your observations. For example, you could create a checklist of things to look for as you observe a certain situation. During your observation, use the checklist to guide your note taking. The checklist and thorough notes add reliability to your observations.

- *Personal experiences.* Some assignments allow you to use information gathered from your own experiences. Just be sure the experiences you draw from are directly related to the topic of your paper. Also, back up your experiences with more objective information from sources you trust, such as reference books or articles in academic journals.

## ORGANIZING YOUR INFORMATION

Index cards are an excellent way to begin organizing your information. Fill out one index card per source, including main ideas and references to page numbers. (You'll need to know page numbers for the bibliography or references part of your paper.)

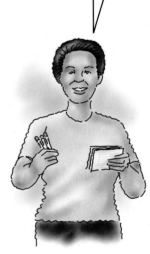

Try using a color-coding system or symbols to keep your index cards organized. Just be creative and use a method that works easily for you.

Start by creating cards for your general sources and then move to more specific sources. This is a good time to take notes on each source and look for quotes as well. Be sure to copy down quotes word for word and cite them accurately on your index cards. In the sources themselves, use sticky notes to mark relevant chapters or sections. For photocopied pages, you can use colorful highlighters to mark important information.

Next, sort your index cards according to topic. If you have several sources that provide the same information, discard the ones you won't need. Begin thinking about the basic layout of your paper at this point. Separate your cards into three stacks:

- The first stack is for information that belongs toward the beginning of your paper.
- The second stack is for material you plan to use toward the middle of your paper.
- The third stack holds the cards you'll need to consult when writing the end of your paper.

## EVALUATING YOUR INFORMATION

After you've organized your sources, you'll need to check each one for relevance to your topic:

- Check the publication date (if possible, try to avoid using sources published more than 5 years ago).
- Make sure each source contains supporting information.

If you find a source that argues against your thesis, it may still be relevant to your paper. You can write a stronger paper by including differing points of view and defending your thesis. Sources that contain counterpoint material also help you determine how well your thesis holds up against arguments. If you find that your thesis is too weak, this is a good point in the writing process to rethink the focus of your paper. It would be much easier to rewrite your thesis than it would be to try to write an entire paper about an idea you're unable to support.

Once you've sorted relevant sources, make sure the information they contain is reliable. As you review each source, ask yourself:

- *Is the author biased?* Does the author merely present personal opinions without backing up statements with facts or research? Does the author criticize certain ideas without giving solid reasons why those ideas are faulty? Have statistics been presented in a misleading way to further the author's opinion?

- *Is the source primary or secondary?* A primary source contains firsthand information. A secondary source restates material from a primary source. Occasionally, secondary sources reproduce quotes made in primary sources. Out of context, those quotes may take on different meanings, which affect their reliability. Whenever possible, use primary sources.

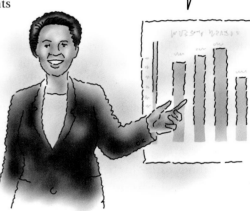

*Remember that statistics can be manipulated. Even if information is presented as fact, you still need to evaluate it!*

After evaluating your sources, keep only those that contain reliable information important to your topic. Then, set aside those index cards for sources you've decided not to use. Later, when you're sure you're not going to need those sources, you can discard them.

## CREATING AN OUTLINE

The next stage in the writing process is creating an outline. Your thesis statement can serve as the outline's introduction. This will help you stay focused on your main point as you write the rest of the outline. Another way to stay focused is to write a brief conclusion. You can expand this conclusion later when you write the first draft of your paper.

Next, refer to your index card notes as you map out the body of the outline. If you're required to submit a title page, table of contents, appendix, or bibliography with your final paper, use simple one-line entries to note these items on your outline as well.

When deciding how to organize the body of your outline, think about your three stacks of index cards for the beginning, middle, and end.

As you write your outline, and even as you write your paper, you're free to move sections around and reorganize information. The purpose of having an outline is to give yourself a guide. But it isn't set in stone. An outline allows you to see the organization of your paper at a glance and make necessary changes before you begin writing your first draft.

---

## Anatomy of an Outline

**TIPS from THE PROS**

Follow these tips when creating an outline for your paper.
I. Creating an outline
   A. Sections
      1. Introduction (use thesis statement)
      2. Body (consult index cards)
      3. Conclusion
      4. Other items (one-line entries)
         a. title page
         b. table of contents
         c. appendix
         d. bibliography
   B. Organization
      1. Use index cards to organize info in the body
         a. beginning of paper (first stack of cards)
         b. middle of paper (second stack of cards)
         c. end of paper (third stack of cards)
      2. Move sections around as necessary

---

## WRITING A FIRST DRAFT

The first draft of your paper is just that—a draft. Don't worry about editing and polishing your writing at this point. There will be plenty of time for that later. The most important thing is to put your ideas into sentences and paragraphs.

While writing the first draft, you'll develop the introduction and body of your paper. You'll need to begin keeping track of references (using footnotes or the system required by your instructor) and bibliography sources. You'll also expand on the brief conclusion you wrote for your outline.

Another important part of writing a first draft involves developing the tone you'll use throughout your paper. To do this, think about your audience:

- Is this paper intended for your instructor?

- Will you be presenting it to the rest of the class?

To have a consistent tone in all sections of your paper, keep your audience in mind as you write.

Your outline should guide the process of writing the first draft. As you begin writing, however, feel free to make changes if the organization of your outline isn't working. Using a word processing program makes it easy to move sections of text. Just remember to save your work often! It's also a good idea to back up your writing on disk or by some other method.

The last step in writing your first draft is to put it away for a while. Depending on your schedule, this may mean 24 hours or several days. This gives your brain time to process what you've written. During the time you spend away from writing, you may think of ways to improve your paper. Whether you come up with the perfect introduction or a better way to state your conclusion, these ideas are valuable. Write them down so you can incorporate them later as you make revisions to your first draft.

> The wheels in your head will keep turning even after you take a break from your paper. After you finish the first draft, put it away for a while and let your brain keep working.

## REVISING THE FIRST DRAFT

After you've been away from your paper for some time, you can begin revising for the second draft. By this time, you should have a better idea of how the overall organization of your paper is working. If any big organizational changes need to be made, such as moving one whole section closer to the beginning or the end of the paper, now is the time to make them.

Again, if you're working on a computer, remember to save often! Another helpful tip for computer users is to rename each draft (e.g., Draft 1, Draft 2, Draft 3). That way, you can always refer to a previous version of your paper if you delete a section by mistake or if you decide to go back to your original organization.

With each draft, your paper should resemble more closely how it will look in its final stage. But how many drafts are needed? Reading your entire paper aloud is one way to help you notice parts that may need improvement. As you read, consider the following:

- *Organization*. Does the overall organization make sense? Does the paper move forward in a logical and clear way?

- *Paragraph structure*. Does each paragraph have a main idea and supporting details? Does the paper include transitions from one paragraph to the next?

- *Sentence flow*. Do the sentences flow smoothly from one to the next?

As you revise your paper, also keep the due date in mind. Be sure to allow yourself enough time for editing the final draft.

Once you're satisfied with the body of your paper, it's time to create the title page, table of contents (page numbers can be inserted after your final edit), bibliography and references, appendix, and any other items required by your instructor. Then, have someone else read the paper—it's always a good idea to have a fresh pair of eyes look for anything you may have missed. (Your school may also have a writing center staffed with people who can fill this role.) Your reviewer can look at things such as spelling, grammar, organization, logic, and any other elements your instructor may use to grade the paper. But keep in mind that any suggestions made by your reviewer are merely suggestions. In the end, you must decide yourself what changes to make.

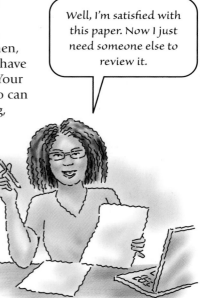

*Well, I'm satisfied with this paper. Now I just need someone else to review it.*

## FINALIZING THE PAPER

The final stage in the writing process involves editing, formatting, and proofreading your paper.

1. During editing, it's helpful to consult other resources, such as a dictionary, thesaurus, and an English grammar and usage guide. These resources should be available in the reference section of the library. As you edit your work, follow these guidelines.

   - Check the paper's tone to make sure it remains consistent.

   - Make sure terms are used consistently throughout the paper. For example, if you used *congestive heart failure* in one paragraph, avoid changing it to *heart failure* in another paragraph if it refers to the same condition.

   - Spell check your paper. Check any words the spell-checker doesn't recognize (such as scientific terms). Remember that the spell-checker doesn't know the difference between "your" and "you're"—and can leave you with many confusing errors.

   - Check your grammar. For example, make sure all singular subjects have singular verbs and all plural subjects have plural verbs. ("He walks," not "He walk.")

   - Check your punctuation. All sentences should end with a period or other punctuation mark. All text in quotes should have both opening and closing quotation marks.

   - Check the spacing between lines of text. Most instructors require students to use double spacing to allow plenty of room for marks and comments.

   - Make sure the font size is appropriate (12-pt. font is standard).

2. The next step in finalizing your paper is formatting. Use the following tips as you format your paper:

- Follow your instructor's formatting guidelines. If specific guidelines aren't provided, your instructor may require you to adhere to a particular style manual instead (such as the *Publication Manual of the American Psychological Association*). Style manuals can answer questions you may have about specialized terms and industry style and formatting standards. The manual will likely also include information on how to format your references and bibliography. These resources also can be found in the reference section of the library.

- Print a hard copy of your paper. Reviewing a hard copy is easier than looking at your paper on a computer screen and formatting errors are much more visible.

3. Take a short break before you begin the last step—proofreading. If you're too familiar with the text of your paper, your eyes might begin to skip over errors. By waiting a bit, you'll come back refreshed and ready to read your paper closely. Here are some proofreading tips:

- Read your entire paper aloud (if possible).

- Remember your spell-checker will miss common errors and may actually create errors—you need to check every word yourself.

- Be on the lookout for any errors in punctuation or capitalization.

- When you come across an unfamiliar word, look it up in the dictionary to check its spelling and meaning.

- Read your paper from end to beginning. It sounds strange, but this will interrupt the rhythm you've developed from reading your paper many times and will help you see errors you might otherwise miss.

After completing this last step, you can hand in your final paper feeling confident about your work!

# RESEARCHING FOR WRITING OR PRESENTATIONS

As mentioned previously, you'll likely need to do some research for writing a paper or preparing a class presentation. Your best methods of research are your school's library and the Internet.

# Library Research

Many younger students have grown up with computers and the Internet and seldom use libraries. Don't fall into this trap! Libraries continue to provide a wide range of valuable information, much of which cannot be found online. Get to know your school's library. It likely has an online catalog that makes it easy to search for the information you need. Specific library resources typically include:

- Books and journals stored in the library stacks, reference room, and other reading rooms. Especially important are the journals of the professional associations in your chosen health career.

- Reference manuals, indexes of articles sorted by subject and title, and other specialized works kept in the reference department.

- Librarians—yes, people! Librarians are highly trained experts on research techniques, as well as the information that can be found in the library. They will be happy to give you personal assistance if you experience any difficulty finding material on your topic.

# Internet Research

When you sit down at a computer, you literally have access to a world of resources. The material you can find online far outweighs the volume of material stored in any library. The key is determining which sources on the Web are reliable and which are not.

## WEBSITES

Websites consist of one or more Web pages. When you are "surfing the Web," it means you are moving from one Web page to another. You do this by clicking on hyperlinks, which usually look like graphics, buttons, or underlined words onscreen.

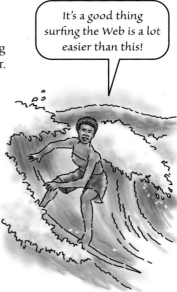

*It's a good thing surfing the Web is a lot easier than this!*

All websites have a "home page." This is the main page for the site. A home page usually includes text or graphics as well as links to additional pages within the site. Because there are billions of websites on the Internet, it's helpful to have an idea of how to search for particular information and which websites to trust. By following some simple guidelines, your online research will go more smoothly.

### On the Corner of http:// and www

Each Web page has an address, otherwise known as a URL (universal resource locator). If you know a site's URL, you'll have no trouble locating it among the many other sites on the Web.

Web addresses, especially lengthy ones, might look confusing. But each address is made up of the same basic components. Below is an explanation of each component, based on the fictional Web address http://www.acmesportsequipment.com.

- *http://* These letters stand for hypertext transfer protocol. Most Web addresses start out this way.
- *www.* This acronym for World Wide Web appears in many, but not all, URLs.
- *acmesportsequipment* This portion of the Web address indicates the name of the site. In this example, the site is named for the Acme Sports Equipment Company.
- *.com* This portion of the URL is called the suffix. The suffix provides additional information about the site.

### What's in a Name?

Usually, you can gather certain information about a website just by looking at the suffix of its URL. Here's a list of common suffixes:

- *.com* This suffix usually indicates that a particular site is intended for commercial use. Most sites ending in .com are owned by businesses or individuals.
- *.edu* Web addresses ending in .edu indicate educational institutions (colleges and universities). If your school has a website, its URL probably ends in .edu.
- *.gov* This suffix indicates that a particular site is owned and operated by a government institution or agency.
- *.net* Web addresses ending in .net usually indicate Internet service providers (ISPs).
- *.org* This suffix indicates a nonprofit organization.

## THE SEARCH IS ON!

What happens if you don't know the URL of the site you're looking for? Or what if you prefer to search for several different websites that deal with a specific topic? This is where search engines come in.

For example, suppose you needed to locate information on how to perform cardiopulmonary resuscitation (CPR). You use a search engine such as Google and enter keywords into the search box. For this particular search, *CPR* would be an appropriate keyword. The search engine then compiles a list of websites that may be relevant to your search. You view the results of your search and click on the links to websites that seemed applicable.

Most Web browsers now have one or more search engines, such as Google or Yahoo, built in on a toolbar for easy searching. Or you can go directly to a search engine's site, such as www.google.com or www.yahoo.com

## Improve Your Searching Skills

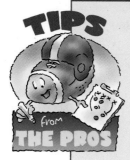

With so much information on the Web, it's sometimes tricky trying to locate the information you need. The following tips will help you perform better Internet searches.

### Starting Your Search

- Avoid using words such as *a, an,* and *the* when entering keywords into a search bar. Most search engines ignore these words anyway.
- If you are looking for a specific phrase, enclose it in quotation marks. Most search engines recognize text contained within quotes as a single item. For example, if you needed to find information on heart disease in children, you would enter *"heart disease in children"* in the search bar.
- Be specific. Entering *diabetes education* in the search bar would give you more specific results to sort through than the more general search term *diabetes*.
- Avoid being overly specific. If your search returns very few results, broaden your search terms.

### Keeping At It

- If your first search is unsuccessful, try rephrasing your keyword(s). You may find what you need by looking up a related word.
- If you still can't find what you're looking for, try using a different search engine.
- For complicated searches, look for an "advanced search" button in the search engine. Advanced search features include the ability to exclude results with a certain key term and to search for synonyms in addition to an exact phrase.

Again, don't forget the librarians! If you still have trouble with your searches after trying these techniques, a librarian may be able to help you find what you're looking for.

## THE RELIABILITY TEST

Just because information has been posted on the Internet doesn't make it trustworthy. When performing research online, remember to be wary of unreliable websites. Use these tips when trying to spot the difference between reliable and unreliable sites:

- Compare sources to verify information. If a statement posted on a website seems too outrageous to be true, check it against a source you trust.
- Beware of sites that seem biased or push a specific agenda. These sites may skew facts or give blatant misinformation.
- Pay attention to URL suffixes. Usually, you can assume that sites ending in .gov or .edu contain reliable information. However, be wary of .edu sites that are owned by individual students at a university. These sites generally are not regulated for accuracy.

- As a general rule, the sites of well-known associations or agencies tend to post reliable information.
- Be especially critical of information posted on sites owned by individuals or small, unknown organizations. The owners of these sites do not have the same accountability as reputable businesses or organizations.

> When conducting online research, only use information from sites you can trust.

## Reliable Websites

Your instructor may be able to provide you with a more complete listing of reliable health professions websites related to your specific career area. Check the chart for a list to get you started.

| Site Name | Address | Brief Summary |
| --- | --- | --- |
| American Association of Medical Assistants | www.aama-ntl.org | Offers information for students and employers |
| American Dental Assistants Association | www.dentalassistant.org | Includes information on membership in the association, education, and employment |
| American Heart Association | www.americanheart.org | Includes information on continuing education and resources for professionals |
| American Red Cross | www.redcross.org | Offers health and safety information |
| American Society of Radiologic Technologists | www.asrt.org | Includes information on continuing education; provides links to online publications and an on-line learning center |
| HealthAnswers Education | www.healthanswers.com | Offers interactive training for individuals in the pharmaceutical and biotechnology industries |
| Lippincott Williams & Wilkins | www.lww.com | Publisher of allied health texts; provides health care news, continuing education information, and other resources |
| Massage Therapy Foundation | www.massagetherapy foundation.org | Provides resources for students, including a massage therapy research database |

| Site Name | Address | Brief Summary |
|-----------|---------|---------------|
| Mayo Clinic | www.mayoclinic.com | Provides health information from the scientists and doctors at the Mayo Clinic |
| National Institutes of Health (NIH) | www.nih.gov | Government-sponsored site; functions as the home page for all other NIH sites, such as the National Cancer Institute, National Institute on Aging, and others |
| PubMed | http://www.ncbi.nlm .nih.gov/pubmed | A medical information search engine from the National Library of Medicine, useful for professional medical material |
| WebMD | www.webmd.com | Offers health information and links to articles on health-related issues; provides online discussion boards |

# GROUP PROJECTS

When group-writing projects or presentations are assigned, your main focus should be on acting as a dependable teammate. Not only will you need to contribute quality material, but you'll need to offer your input to the rest of the group and complete your work on time.

As described in Chapter 8, study group members need to be *committed contributors* who are *compatible* with one another and *considerate* of each other. The same is true when working with a group of your classmates on a writing assignment or class presentation.

- First and foremost, everyone in the group needs to be committed to the project.
- Each person is responsible for bringing something to the table, such as supplying ideas and written or graphical material.
- Even if your instructor assigned you to work with a group of people you don't get along with, you should find a way to overlook your differences and focus on the project.
- If everyone in the group makes an effort to speak politely and be considerate of each other's time, the project will go more smoothly.

# Be a Team Player

When working in a group on a writing assignment or class presentation, the group uses the same process as described earlier for preparing a presentation or the writing process. Group dynamics, however, often require call for additional planning and shared responsibilities. Keep these guidelines in mind:

> Be a team player when helping out with group projects!

1. Schedule a group meeting as soon as possible to get started. Don't let anyone put things off. Explain that you're too busy and won't have time at the last minute to do your share.

2. Begin your first meeting by brainstorming together about the written assignment's topic or the presentation's audience and goals. Make sure everyone understands the assignment and is on the same wavelength. Then discuss who should do what. One or more students may begin research and gathering information, another may do the initial drafting, others may develop visual aids, and so on. You also need a team leader—someone to keep everyone on schedule, organize meetings, etc. The team leader needs good social skills and the ability to motivate cooperation among everyone in the group.

3. Assigned tasks can then be carried out individually, but everyone should stay in touch. For example, a student developing visual aids should be talking to those doing the researching and drafting to see what visuals will be needed or useful.

4. Before writing the first draft or outlining the presentation, the group should meet again to go over the work in process. Everyone should be comfortable with the plan as it has emerged so far. At this time, make final decisions about who will complete the next stages, such as who will do the presenting or final editing. With a presentation involving multiple speakers, plan for the student with the strongest speaking skills to open and/or close the presentation, with others doing specific parts in the middle.

5. The whole group should work together during the presentation practice or revising of the paper. Everyone should have the opportunity to comment on polishing the final work.

6. With a presentation, especially if technology is used for visual aids, one student should manage the visuals while one or more others do the presenting. If several students present different segments, plan transitions so that the presentation flows without pauses or delays.

# COMPUTER COMMUNICATION

Two common forms of computerized communication use the Internet and email. All the same principles of communication generally apply the same as with written and spoken communication, with a few additional considerations.

## On the Web

Because the Internet connects computers around the world, it is easily used by many as a communication tool. Here are few examples:

- The Web allows businesses to communicate with each other and with consumers.
- Health care providers use the Internet to communicate with each other and patients or the general public.
- Students can use the Internet to communicate with classmates and instructors.

A traditional method of online communication uses online message boards, or discussion boards, where you can post questions or comments to your classmates and instructors. Some message boards are set up so students and instructors from different schools anywhere in the world can communicate with each other. Because their format encourages discussion, message boards can be a great source of supplemental material.

Nowadays, it is very easy to access the Internet through wired or wireless connections available at school, in public "hot spots," in many homes, and on many mobile phones. Most computers already include the appropriate hardware and software. Through programs such as Skype, you can also have direct video conferencing between two computers equipped with Web cams, speakers, and microphones. Other online meeting services allow video to be sent out from a presenter and multiple viewers to connect back with the full group through audio or text messages.

New applications for online communication are being implemented almost every day, and the specific forms you may use now as a student and in your future health career may vary. The use of these programs is increasingly simple—and now can usually be learned in a few minutes.

More important, however, is recognizing that even these forms of communication, which may seem as casual as a telephone call between friends, require professionalism. Always assume that what you say or write online might be captured or saved and then viewed later by someone else. Speak or write in respectful tones and maintain the privacy and confidentiality of others.

*Technology keeps getting easier and more available, but common courtesy never goes out of style!*

# Email

*Email* is now a preferred form of communication in education, business, and many health care practices. In addition to messages, you can send documents and digital images to anyone with Internet access. If you have a free email account through your school or place of employment, it's a good idea to keep it separate from your personal account. This will help keep you and your school materials organized!

## Email Best Practices

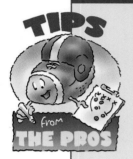

Email communication with an instructor or business associate is a professional form of communication and shouldn't look like the sort of messages frequently sent between friends. For example, rather than using abbreviations and shorthand, most instructors expect email messages to be in full sentences with correctly spelled words and reasonable grammar. Follow these guidelines:

- Use a professional email name, not a casual or humorous name you might use with friends. For example, JohnSmith@gmail.com is better than SuperGuy@gmail.com.

- In the subject line, label your message so the reader knows at a glance what the message concerns. "May I make an appointment?" is clear, but "In your office now?" isn't.

- Address email messages as you would a letter, such as "Dear Professor Jones." Be sure to sign with your full name.

- Get to your point quickly and concisely. Don't force the reader to scroll ahead down a long email to see what you want to say.

- Avoid any temptations to be funny, ironic, sarcastic, etc. Write as you would in a paper for class. In a large lecture class or an online course, your email voice may be the primary way your instructor knows you, and emotionally charged messages can be confusing or give a poor impression.

- Don't use capital letters to emphasize. All caps look like SHOUTING.

- Avoid abbreviations, nonstandard spelling, slang, and emoticons like smiley faces. These are not professional.

- When replying to a message, leave the original message within yours (typically below your new message). Your reader may need to recall what he or she said in the original message.

- Be polite. End the message with a "Thank you" or something similar.

- Check the subject line and text of your message for correct spelling and punctuation. Many email programs include a spell-check feature—use it!

- Review your message for content as well as correctness before clicking to send it. You may have expressed an emotion or thought that you will think better about later.

# Communicating in Online Courses

Many schools now offer online courses you can take from the comfort of your own home. Such courses can include most of the elements from traditional classes, such as instructor-led presentations, question-and-answer sessions, assignments, and tests. Online courses are especially convenient for working students who have limited time to come to campus. However, online courses require high levels of commitment and self-discipline. Students take more responsibility for their own learning.

Before deciding to take an online course, think about your individual strengths and weaknesses as well as your personal learning style:

> *I never thought I'd take an online course, but I've found it plays to my strengths!*

- Are you self-disciplined?
- Do you enjoy being able to complete tasks according to your own schedule?
- Do you need the structure of a traditional classroom course?
- Online courses typically require a lot of reading and independent study—does that match your learning style?

An additional consideration with online courses involves communication with the instructor and sometimes with other students. Unlike regular classes where you hear others speak and can talk directly to your instructor and ask questions or meet during office hours, your communication in an online course will be mostly, or entirely, written. Are you comfortable with written communication and confident of your ability to express yourself well in writing? If you feel you need more experience with academic writing, you might choose to put off taking any online courses until you've done more writing assignments in regular courses and have gained that confidence.

A final word: because most or all of the communication with an online instructor will occur through email, be sure to follow the guidelines listed in *Best Email Practices*. Your instructor may never even see your face—the impression you make will come entirely from your words!

## CHAPTER SUMMARY

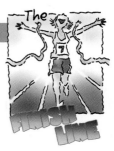

- Improve your ability to express yourself by speaking up during class and participating in discussions.
- Develop good writing skills now for your future use in health care settings, such as writing accurate and concise reports in patient charts.
- Use the library, Internet, and other resources to research information for written assignments and class presentations.

- Be a dependable team player in group-writing projects or class presentations. Participate by giving your input, completing your work on time, and being sure to contribute quality material.
- Use effective techniques in all forms of academic and professional communication, including online and email practices.

## REVIEW QUESTIONS

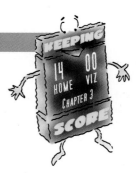

1. What specific things can you do to overcome stage fright when preparing to give a presentation to a class?
2. When gathering material for a paper, what are several sources where you can look to find information?
3. Why is it important to follow the full process steps for a writing assignment or presentation?
4. Name three important things to remember when working on a team project.
5. Describe the appearance of a professional email.

## CHAPTER ACTIVITIES

1. Group Discussion: Begin with a warm-up exercise to get everyone participating. Think of something, aside from family and friends, that you value (such as a painting, CD collection, book, etc.). Then, in 1 to 2 minutes, share with the rest of the class what that object is and why it's important to you. After everyone has had a chance to participate in the warm-up exercise, discuss as a group several reasons why people may have a fear of public speaking. Why is the ability to speak up particularly important in a health care setting?

2. Online Investigation: Visit your school's website to learn whether you may include online courses as part of your academic program. (If not, for this exercise, go to the website of a nearby community college or state university.) Choose a course you might find interesting and learn as much about it as you can. How is information presented (videos, textbook, online instruction)? What are the major kinds of assignments? Is there an opportunity to meet online with other students? What kinds of communications with the instructor are expected? Finally, based on what you learn about this course, decide whether you are prepared with the right skills at present for succeeding in this course.

## CHAPTER 8

# Study Skills

*On completion of this chapter and the learning activities you will be able to:*

- Use course materials to focus on your study goals
- Select and prepare a study space
- Improve your concentration and memorization skills
- Explore different study strategies to improve your efficiency
- Build and use a study group effectively
- Make use of supplemental study materials
- Improve your study skills for math and science

Much of your time as a student will be spent studying. If that thought makes you groan, don't despair! There are many simple strategies you can use to make the most of your study time and the resources available to you. In this chapter, you'll learn how to study effectively, starting with how to select a study space and how to prepare yourself for studying. You'll learn tips for improving your concentration and long-term memory as well. Study strategies can help you make the most of your time to help ensure your success as a student. In addition, you'll learn how to form and work with a study group and how to use textbook and other resources as you study. Finally, you'll learn some special study skills for math and science.

## WHAT ARE YOU GOING TO STUDY?

Although it may seem obvious, you need a focus before starting to study. Are you studying a chapter to prepare for class? Studying for an upcoming test? Studying how to perform a certain health care procedure before you do it in the lab tomorrow? Start by considering your reasons for studying and setting your goals.

This step begins with materials your instructor has provided you, including:

- the syllabus
- study guides and lecture outlines
- practice exercises
- assignment instructions

## Start with the Syllabus

Chapter 2 points out the importance of the syllabus for each class and how to use it. The syllabus gives you key information such as reading assignments, exam dates, and due dates for papers and other out-of-class work. Chapter 2 also discusses how to manage your time well by scheduling study periods well ahead of time to avoid last-minute "cramming," which is the least effective way to study. Your syllabus is your road map for starting to get organized for studying, but it's not your only resource.

## Study Guides and Lecture Outlines

Many instructors not only tell you what general topic you'll cover each day of class, but they may also provide an outline of each day's lecture for you. You can use this outline as you prepare for class. It allows you to focus your reading and studying on the points listed in the outline. Keep these main ideas in mind as you read to help you prepare well for class.

An added benefit is that you will not have to take as many notes during class because the outline is already provided for you! And don't forget to put the study guide or outline in your notebook under a tab where you can find it later. You'll also find it very helpful when studying for tests.

## Practice Exercises

Some instructors also provide practice exercises for you. These may be on a handout or on the course website. Practice exercises are a great way to drill. If your instructor goes to the trouble of giving you practice exercises for a chapter or section, you should assume that the material is particularly important to know and that it may be on a test. File these exercises in a safe place so you can use them later as you study. Save any completed exercises so you can check your work when you get graded tests back.

*Doing drills and practice exercises is a great way to prepare for upcoming tests!*

## Assignment Instructions

Your instructor may also give you a handout that tells you exactly how certain assignments are to be done. These instructions can include things such as:

- style guides for papers—details on how papers should be typed, how to format your citations and bibliography, what margins to use, etc.
- step-by-step walkthroughs—such as for clinical procedures; sometimes, many different procedures start with the same basic steps
- research tips—resources for finding information on the Internet or in the library

Remember to file your assignment instructions in your notebook under the correct tab.

# GETTING ORGANIZED TO STUDY

Studying is much more efficient when you're organized. Organization is a key to your success not only as a health professions student, but also as a health care professional. Being organized for studying simply makes the most efficient use of your time.

If you're already a very organized person, you may not need to make any changes in your system for keeping track of things. On the other hand, if you consider yourself less than organized or even hopelessly disorganized, take heart! The following tips and suggestions are simple and easy to implement.

> Organization is a key to your success both as a student and as a future health care professional.

## Location, Location, Location

The first step to getting organized is finding or making a place for everything. This means you'll need to find a place to keep the materials and supplies for each class you're taking. Most students find that the best organizational system uses three-ring binders (or twin-pocket folders with notebook fasteners) with tabbed dividers.

Dedicate one binder for each class. Keep all handouts, notes, charts—everything related to that class—together in that binder.

## Divide and Conquer

Next, decide how you want to organize the material in each binder, using labeled tabbed dividers or a similar system. You may find it helpful to use the same set of divider names in each binder. This will minimize the time it takes to find things. Use a pen or colored permanent marker to label the tabs on the dividers. You can purchase tabbed dividers or make your own from card-stock paper. The following is an example of a typical set of divider names:

- schedule
- syllabus
- handouts
- assignments
- notes

In this system, your class schedule is at the front. This helps you see at a glance what's going to be covered in the next class period. The syllabus needs to be accessible, too, because it contains other critical information. Every time you receive a new handout, place it behind the "Handouts" tab; do the same with assignments. The last section is for taking notes in class and during your reading. Keep a supply of new notebook paper behind this tab.

---

### Organizing Your Notes

You may prefer to use a spiral notebook instead of loose-leaf paper for taking notes. Just be sure to keep the notebook with the appropriate binder for each class. To avoid confusion, use a separate notebook for each class. Mixing notes from several classes will disrupt your organization and derail your game plan.

Chapter 6 describes how to take good notes in class. After class, take a few minutes to organize your notes by following these simple steps.

- Record the date of the lecture.
- Number your pages.
- Write down reminders about upcoming assignments and due dates. Make sure the dates are written in your weekly planner.

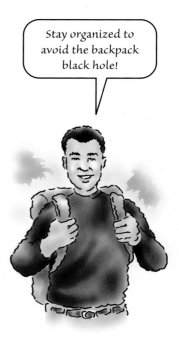

*Stay organized to avoid the backpack black hole!*

## The Backpack Black Hole

One final note about organization: Beware the backpack black hole. If you are in a rush after class, it may be tempting to gather your papers, shove them into your backpack, and forget about them. The only problem with this method is that when you need to review one of those papers several days or weeks later, you might not be able to find it. A lack of organization makes it easy for important papers to get lost. The backpack black hole occurs when things go in and are never to be seen again.

# STUDYING 101

Studying seems simple: Get out your books and notes and study them. But what does it really mean to study? Studying involves:

- refreshing your memory
- taking in new information
- organizing and memorizing data

That's a lot! It's no surprise that many students sit down to study and find themselves feeling overwhelmed. And then any little distraction can throw a wrench in the works, keeping you from studying efficiently. That's why it's important to study the right way.

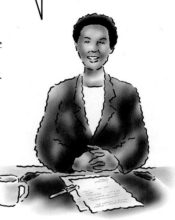

> When it comes to studying, think **location, location, location!** Finding a good place to study is just as important as the study methods you use.

## Scope out a Study Area

First, find a good place to study. Look for a location that is free of distractions. (See *How to Find a Distraction-Free Study Zone.*) Make sure the area is large enough for you to arrange all your study materials. Think about any furniture you might need, such as a desk or large table.

Many students prefer to sit at a table when they study. This arrangement keeps them alert and focused while helping them keep their materials organized. They can put the study materials they're using on the table and keep materials they'll need later underneath it. Other students feel more comfortable sitting on a sofa, with their study materials on a coffee table or spread out on the floor below. One place you may want to avoid studying is your bed, which may tempt you to take a nap!

## How to Find a Distraction-Free Study Zone

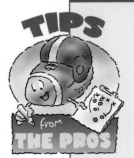

Think about two or three areas that might make good study spaces. Then choose the place that best addresses these questions:

- Are there a lot of other people in the same space who could interrupt me?
- Are there things in the space that will distract me from studying?
- Is there a TV or radio in the space that might be turned on?
- Is there a phone that might ring too often?
- Is this space easy for me to get to on a regular basis?
- Is the temperature comfortable? If it isn't, can I change it?
- Will cooking odors come into this space, making me feel hungry and distracted?
- Is this space big enough so it won't get cluttered when I spread out all my materials?
- Is there enough light so I can read without straining my eyes?

## LIGHTING

Make sure your study space has good lighting you can control. Light is very important. Too much will make your eyes hurt, whereas too little will make your eyes strain. The light should shine evenly over all your work and not directly into your eyes.

## TEMPERATURE

You'll want to be comfortable when you study. Being too cold will distract you; it's difficult to take notes with cold fingers. Being too warm also can hurt your accuracy, speed, and mental sharpness— plus it makes you sleepy! For good studying, the best temperature is between 65° and 70° F (18° to 21° C).

To make sure your study space is a comfortable temperature, test out a few spaces. Sit down and read or study for a half hour. Are you under an air-conditioning or heating vent that will make you too cold or too hot? Are you near a door that causes a draft whenever it's opened? These factors are out of your control and should disqualify a potential study space.

## SURROUNDINGS

Your study space should be inviting. You should feel good about yourself when you're there. A pleasant space can make you more alert. Here are some tips for improving your study surroundings:

- The right kind of background music can promote relaxed alertness, which stimulates learning. It also may improve your recall. In theory, if you always study biology with Bach in the background, you'll remember biology facts when you hear Bach. But be careful with music that is too loud or that will tempt you to sing along.

- Let the answering machine or voice mail pick up your calls, ideally in another room.

- Turn off the TV (or better yet, study in a room without a TV).

- Some people like white noise: a bubbling aquarium, quiet instrumental music, or even an electric fan. White noise blocks out other sounds without creating a distraction.

## Pregame Stretch

Your brain is part of your body. If your body is uncomfortable, your brain has a harder time doing its work. When you're studying, you need your brain to focus on your work, not your aching back. You can stay comfortable by having good posture, avoiding eyestrain, moving around, and eating healthy snacks during long study sessions. (See *Fit for Studying.*)

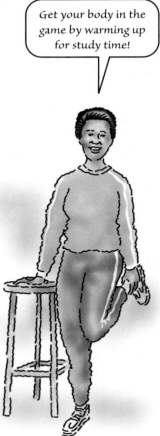

*Get your body in the game by warming up for study time!*

**Fit For Studying**

Here are some ways to stay alert and be comfortable as you study.

- Sit up straight to keep your back and neck from getting stiff. It's worth the effort and it can become a habit if you stick with it. Sitting up straight also keeps you alert and helps you concentrate.

- Position your reading material at a 45-degree angle from your work surface at least 15 inches away from your eyes. If you're too close, your eyes can't focus properly. If you're too far away, you'll strain forward.

- Don't be afraid to get up and walk around every so often when you're studying. Stay in your study area, but try pacing around, doing jumping jacks, or performing simple stretching exercises. When you stand, 5% to 15% more blood flows to your brain. This means your brain gets more oxygen and is more stimulated!

- What about food? If you're going to study for more than an hour at a time, bring a healthy and easy snack, like grapes, so you can eat without mess or distraction.

## The Whistle: Getting Started

Sometimes, it's easier to find a good study space than to actually sit down in that space and study! Getting started can be a big challenge.

The first step in meeting that challenge is planning ahead. Decide which tasks you want to accomplish before you sit down to study and develop a plan for accomplishing those tasks. As mentioned previously, start with your syllabus and other course materials to get focused. The next step is breaking your big tasks down into smaller tasks. Several small tasks will be easier to accomplish than one big task. With each accomplishment, you'll become more confident, which will motivate you to keep going!

### HAVE A GAME PLAN

Before you start a study session, plan it out. Have a goal for each session and a game plan for achieving that goal. Ask yourself the following questions.

- What do I want to get out of this study time?

- What do I need to learn from the material?

Skim the material you need to study and decide how much of it you'll really need to dive deep into and how much you can cover with just a few notes. Not everything needs detailed attention. That way, you'll spend your time wisely and get more out of studying.

## TIMING IS EVERYTHING

Choose your study time carefully. Try not to set aside time you usually spend eating or socializing for studying; you'll only think about what you're missing. This can be hard to do when you're a busy working student with a family. You might feel that you don't have any time when nothing else important is going on! But there probably are adjustments you can make to your daily routine. For example, if you usually spend 2 hours watching TV after dinner, try spending just 1 hour watching TV and use that other hour for studying.

Also, you should try to study when you are naturally more productive and awake. Some of us are morning people; others are night owls. If you tend to feel fresh and alert in the mornings, consider planning some of your study time then. If you're groggy and tired in the morning, but come alive when the sun goes down, evenings are probably the best time for you to study. Use your planner, as described in Chapter 2, to plan out your study sessions at your best times throughout the week.

## SET ATTAINABLE GOALS

Breaking up big tasks is part of setting attainable goals. When you set realistic goals, you set yourself up for success. By taking small steps toward your ultimate goal, you get moving, which is the most important thing.

For example, suppose you have a reading assignment that you don't feel like starting. Begin by telling yourself that you'll read for just 5 minutes, so at least you can get some of the assignment done. After the first 5 minutes, tell yourself that you'll keep reading for a few more minutes and keep repeating this cycle. Before you know it, you'll have read for a half hour or more and maybe even completed a good portion of the assignment.

## GET YOUR BRAIN IN STUDY MODE

Here are some more questions to ask yourself before and during study time to get your brain into study mode. These questions will help enhance your study time retention and later recall.

- Why is this information important?
- What does this information tell me about other topics?
- Is this information fact or opinion?

- What if I looked at this material in a different way?
- How can I compare and contrast different information?
- Does this material remind me of something else I've learned?

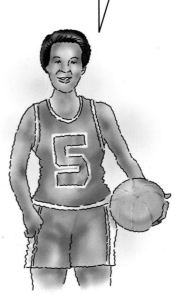

Learning to tune out distractions helps your concentration. Think of a basketball player tuning out a stadium full of people to make a foul shot!

## Improve Your Concentration

We've already talked a little about the distractions that can interfere with your study time. External distractions, like smells or noises, can cause you to lose your concentration. There are internal distractions as well, like hunger or anxiety, that can make studying difficult.

You can learn to improve your concentration skills so you can overcome those distractions. But it takes motivation to improve your concentration. You must want to learn the material in front of you. You have to know why it's important to your future career. Your desire to learn will help you stay focused on studying. Also, you need to be awake, alert, and prepared to learn. Being alert the first time you study helps you avoid multiple review sessions.

As an added bonus, improving your concentration during study time also helps you remember more material. This means you'll get better scores on tests, quizzes, and assignments.

### Do You Have a Wandering Mind?

Some people seem to remember everything they see or hear. Other people forget their own phone numbers. Does your mind wander? To find out how well you pay attention, ask yourself the following questions. If you answer *yes* often, you may have a wandering mind that could use some concentration strategies.

- Do you forget the names of people you just met?
- Do you ask people to repeat themselves?
- Do you lose track of what's going on around you?
- Do you sometimes stare blankly at a page?
- Do you sometimes feel like you don't remember information you just read?

It's normal for your mind to wander occasionally. But the most important thing is being aware of when it happens, so you can get back on track.

## READY YOUR MIND AND BODY

First, you'll need to prepare your mind and body to concentrate. The following strategies will help you find your focus before you begin studying:

- Take a walk for 5 to 10 minutes to clear your head and relax your body.
- Meditate for about 5 minutes. Sit quietly, perhaps in your study area with the lights off. Sit up straight and picture something still and peaceful. Breathe deeply and slowly.
- Try to avoid caffeine. Too much can cause you to become jumpy and make it harder to concentrate.

## CONCENTRATE!

Next, work on improving your concentration as you study. You can do this by using some of the strategies discussed earlier in this chapter, such as avoiding distractions and setting realistic goals. Here are some other good ways to improve your concentration:

- Study during a time of day when you're awake and alert.
- Focus on one topic at a time.
- Keep your brain active by engaging in different activities, such as reading, taking notes, and spending time thinking.
- Take a short break every 45 minutes to 1 hour.

As with so many things, practice makes perfect when it comes to concentration. It might seem discouraging if you get distracted easily the first few times you study. But keep at it and you'll train your brain to stay focused.

# Improve Your Memory Skills

Information is stored in different ways in your brain. That's why it's easy to remember some events or people and harder to remember others. Memory isn't a sense; it's a skill you can develop and improve. By understanding how memory works, you can learn ways to improve it.

## THE MEMORIZATION PROCESS

Why is it that you remember some things but forget others? It depends in large part on how the brain processes memories. The three stages of information processing are:

1. registration
2. short-term memory
3. long-term memory

As you learn new material in school, your goal is to get the most important information into your long-term memory—and then to keep it there. That way, you'll be able to recall what you learned during tests and put your knowledge to use later when you're on the job. Let's take a look at how memories move through the three stages.

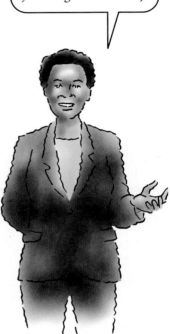

*As a student, one of your main goals is to store important information in your long-term memory.*

## Registration

During registration, the brain receives information. That information eventually may be understood and selected for remembering. Registration is a three-part process: reception, perception, and selection.

1. In the *reception* phase, you automatically take in information, even when not knowing what it means. For instance, you might listen to a patient's bowels and hear whooshing sounds, without knowing what the sounds mean or what condition they represent.

2. During *perception*, you recognize what you've experienced and give it a meaning. Suppose you remember from class that whooshing sounds might mean the bowel is obstructed. You've attached a meaning to the sound—that's perception.

3. Finally, during *selection*, your brain chooses which pieces of information to remember. The information it selects depends on:

   - the information available at the moment
   - your reason for remembering it
   - your background knowledge of the topic
   - the content and how difficult it is
   - the way in which the information is organized

Your brain recognizes information as important or unimportant. If you perceive or decide something is important, like the fact that whooshing sounds could mean an obstructed bowel, then that fact is processed for remembering. If you perceive or decide it's unimportant, the information is forgotten. Processed information is then sent to short-term memory.

## Short-Term Memory

Short-term memory can last as little as 15 seconds—that's short! Short-term memory can't hold very much information and what it can hold doesn't stay there for long. Research has shown that short-term memory can hold five to nine chunks of information, depending on how the information is grouped.

For example, you can remember the numbers 1-9-2-9-0-0-7 by grouping them: 1929 and 007. 1929 is easy to remember because it's a date, and 007 is famous from James Bond movies. This way, instead of trying to remember seven different numbers, you only have to recall two groups of information. Grouping makes space for more data in your short-term memory.

**Break It Up**

When you first learn something new, it's hard for your brain to group the information when it's not sure of relationships among the bits of material. You can make things easier on your brain by learning small chunks of information at a time, instead of trying for one large chunk all at once. Your brain can organize small amounts of information more easily.

### Long-Term Memory

After information has entered short-term memory, your brain either soon forgets it or moves it to long-term memory where it is organized and stored for long periods. How long depends on how completely the information is processed and how often you recall and use it. (See *Making Memories for the Long Haul.*) There are many ways to help move information from short- to long-term memory, but the best way is to recall and use information immediately and often.

## GETTING THINGS INTO YOUR BRAIN: WORKING MEMORY

The term *working memory* describes how your brain stores and retrieves information from short-term and long-term memory. Improving your working memory is critical to remembering what you study. You can use four strategies to improve your working memory:

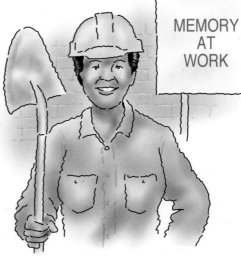

- selection
- association
- organization
- rehearsal

### Selection

During selection, you single out the information you want to remember and start to select ways to process that information. For example, say you need to learn the steps involved in CPR. Because you know you'll need to demonstrate these steps in class, you immediately decide that all the steps are important to remember.

We make more conscious decisions about what is important all the time. For instance, a parent might know the phone number for her child's school or doctor by heart because she made a conscious effort to learn it. Why? Because she decided the number was very important and trained herself to remember it. She selected the number

as information important enough to go into long-term memory.
Learning new material begins with making a conscious decision to
remember it.

## Making Memories for the Long Haul

There are many ways to make sure important information gets into your
long-term memory. Use the following tips while you're studying to help
you identify and sort long-term memory information.

When working alone:

- Attach strong emotions to the material you're studying.
- Rewrite the material in your own words.
- Build a working model of the material you're studying; create an image of it that you can remember.
- Create a song about the material or put definitions to a familiar tune.
- Draw a picture or create a poster using intense colors.
- Repeat and review the material 10 minutes after you read it, 48 hours afterward, and 7 days afterward.
- Summarize the material in your own words in your notes.
- Immediately apply what you've learned to activities in your daily life.
- Use mnemonics and acronyms to organize the material.
- Write about the material in a journal.
- State key information out loud, as though you were lecturing to a group of people.

When working with others:

- Act out the material or role-play a situation related to the material being studied.
- Join a study group or other support group.
- Discuss the information with a peer to gain an additional perspective and solidify the material in your mind.
- Make a videotape or audiotape related to the material being studied.
- Make up and tell a story about the material.

Remember: the more often you think about or repeat a piece of information, the stronger it will be in your short-term memory. Many people
use this technique, for example, to remember the name of someone
they've just met. For example, if you've been introduced to Bob Hall at a
social function, you'll likely still remember his name a week from now

if you use it now in conversation with him, saying things like "That's an interesting idea, Bob." You can also strengthen the memory by associating his name with something else, such as by thinking, "I just met Bob Hall while standing in the hall." It may sound silly, but it works!

### Association

Association is a very powerful way of committing something to memory. It involves making an association between something you already know and the thing you're trying to learn.

For example, to remember information about a particular disease, try associating that information with someone you know who has the disease. This will provide a memory cue that helps you recall the information later.

### Organization

During organization, you memorize information in an ordered way. For example, if it seems there are many steps involved in CPR, break the process down into smaller chunks made up of a few steps each. With repetition, you can push each chunk or group of steps into your long-term memory. Rewrite the steps, recite them out loud, or act them out. This will help you remember the steps more efficiently, move them into long-term memory, and clear your working memory for the next piece of new information.

### Rehearsal

An athlete may practice a certain skill over and over to perfect their technique. Think of a tennis player serving the ball again and again, going through the same motions each time. You can use a similar method to improve your memory skills. Rehearsal involves repeatedly reviewing information you've learned over short periods of time.

Several short bursts of rehearsal are better than one long cram session. For instance, rehearse the steps for CPR for 5 minutes four times a day over 3 days rather than once for an hour. Challenge yourself to rehearse the steps at different times during the day, such as while on the bus ride home, while you're making dinner, or while you're in the shower. Rehearsing information moves it into your long-term memory.

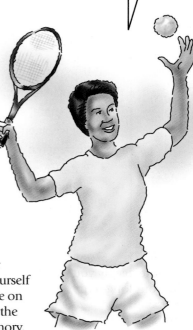

> When it comes to rehearsing information, think of a tennis player practicing their serve over and over. With frequent rehearsal, the information you're trying to remember will become second nature!

## MEMORY RETRIEVAL: USE IT OR LOSE IT

As you have seen, information you process might not stay in your long-term memory if you don't use it regularly. It also can be forgotten if you're not interested in the information, if your purpose for learning is not strong, or if you have few or no connections between the memory and other pieces of information.

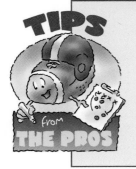

## Hunting Down a Memory

The next time you have trouble remembering something important, try these strategies to search for your lost memory.

1. Say or write down everything you can remember about the information you're seeking.

2. Try to recall events or information in a different order.

3. Re-create the learning environment or relive the event. Include sounds, smells, and details about the weather, objects, or people who were there. Try to recapture what you said, thought, or felt at the time.

### Show Your Interest

In general, the more you care about a topic, the stronger your memory of it will be. For example, if you know you have a quiz next week on a particular topic in anatomy class, you'll store information about that topic more successfully in your long-term memory.

### Understand It

It is possible to memorize information without understanding it. Most of us know the words to the Pledge of Allegiance or the national anthem, even if we might not have thought about what those words really mean. But you have to understand a concept to be able to remember and apply it. Try putting new concepts into your own words and explaining them to someone else. If you can make a layperson understand it, you've got it.

### Go Deep!

The more deeply your brain processes a topic, the more solid your long-term memory of that topic becomes. Processing depth depends on how you process the information, as well as your:

- background knowledge
- desire for learning
- intended use of the information
- level of concentration
- interest in the topic
- overall attitude

> It's easy to remember facts about your favorite sports team. The more interested you are in a topic, the better your retention of it will be.

# Use Study Strategies

There are many study strategies that can help you recall information later during tests and clinical exercises. You've already read about a few of these strategies. Using a variety of study methods helps your brain take in and store the same information in different ways. This creates multiple pathways for your brain to use when you're trying to recall the information later. So give your brain a boost and see which study strategies work best for you!

## PRACTICE, PRACTICE, PRACTICE!

Practice and repetition are very similar to rehearsal. Practice not only helps you store information in your long-term memory, it also helps you retrieve that information from your memory when you need it. Here's how you can apply the strategy of practice and repetition as you study:

- Repeat information out loud or in a group discussion.
- Write or diagram the same material several times.
- Read and then reread information silently.

## TAKE BREAKS

Spaced study is a method that allows you to alternate short study sessions with breaks. Study goals are set by time or task. For example, you could read for at least 15 minutes or read at least 10 pages at a time. After meeting your goal, you would take a short break and then move on to the next goal.

Spaced study works for several reasons:

- It gives immediate rewards for your hard work.
- It helps you complete manageable amounts of work.
- It helps you set deadlines so you can make efficient use of your study time.
- It keeps information moving from your working memory to your long-term memory. (See *Getting Things Into Your Brain: Working Memory*.)
- It gives you study breaks to keep you sharp when you're studying complex subjects.

## MAKE ASSOCIATIONS

Always try to make links between familiar items and new information you want to remember. Once you establish them, these links become automatic. Each time you recall a familiar item, you also remember the information you associated with it.

Follow these steps to form associations as you study:

1. Select the information you want to remember. For example, suppose you want to remember information about osteoporosis, a condition that causes a person's bones to become brittle.

2. Next, create an association to the information. To remember facts about osteoporosis, you might associate that information with a person you know who has the condition. (Osteoporosis reminds me of Mary, who broke her hip. Osteoporosis → Mary → brittle bones.)

The strongest associations are personal, such as associating a song, a person, or a scent with the item you're trying to commit to memory. You probably know certain songs that take you right back to where you were when the song was popular. Associate information to that song and your memory of the information will be just as sharp.

Have fun with it! Use acronyms and acrostics to enhance your long-term memory.

## ACRONYMS AND ACROSTICS

Acronyms and acrostics are handy for recalling information, too. Acronyms are created from the first letter of each item on a list. *ASAP* is an acronym for the phrase "as soon as possible." The acronym *HOMES* helps people remember the Great Lakes:

**H**  Huron

**O**  Ontario

**M**  Michigan

**E**  Erie

**S**  Superior

Acrostics are phrases or sentences that are created from the first letter of each item in a list. In health care, a well-known acrostic is one about the 12 cranial nerves: *On Old Olympus' Towering Tops, A Finn and a Swedish Girl Viewed Some Hops.* This stands for the olfactory, optic, oculomotor, trochlear, trigeminal, abducens, facial, sensorimotor, glossopharyngeal, vagus, spinal accessory, and hypoglossal nerves.

Acronyms and acrostics work in situations where it's hard to find a personal association for a piece of data. (For example, it's difficult to feel personal about the 12 cranial nerves!) Acronyms and acrostics associate key information to a new but easily remembered word or phrase, improving your memory of the information.

## PUT INFORMATION IN ITS PLACE

You can understand a piece of information more easily once you put it in a larger framework of understanding. For example, a small area on a street map makes more sense when you view the map in its entirety. Sometimes, it helps to see how the information you're studying fits into the bigger picture.

You can apply this practice to studying by learning more about a topic in general before focusing on a particular assignment. General magazine articles or Internet encyclopedias are good places to look for general information. After you've gained some background knowledge of a certain topic, you'll be able to associate new information about that topic with what you already know. Your brain can then find a place for the new information in your memory.

## REDUCE INTERFERENCE

Interference sometimes occurs when you're trying to remember two very similar pieces of information. It's like what happens when you tune in one radio station and another station's signal causes static, interfering with your reception. Your brain has to work harder to recognize the differences between the two pieces of information before you can commit both to memory.

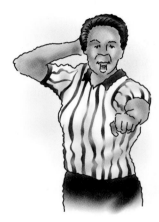

> Interference! Two similar pieces of information may interfere with your brain's ability to remember either of them. Focus on what makes each item different.

For example, if you're trying to learn a lot of new terms and two of them are similar, you might have trouble remembering either of them. To reduce interference, try to relate each new term to information you already know. Your background knowledge will help you recognize the differences between the two terms, allowing you to store each as a separate memory.

If you need to study similar subjects one after the other, take a break between study sessions. Moving to a different study space or changing positions will reinforce the difference between the two subjects. It will associate one subject with one location and the next subject with the next location. This way, your brain can better organize the new information in your memory.

## CREATE LISTS

Lists are another well-known study aid. You can organize ideas by categories that they have in common. The point is that you create a classification system of some kind. Because items relate to each other within the system, you can rearrange and reorganize that information as needed to help your recall.

For example, suppose you're learning about different types of drugs in a pharmacology course. To help you study the material, you create lists of drugs according to what they're used for. Drugs used to treat diabetes are placed in one list, with drugs used to treat heart conditions in another, and so on.

## USE IMAGERY

People often think visually—in images instead of words. Visual aids can help you recall familiar and unfamiliar information when you're studying. This is because images are stored differently than words in the brain.

Adding meaningful doodles, colors, or symbols to your notes allows you to organize them visually by topic. When you use visual representations effectively, you'll remember more information with less effort.

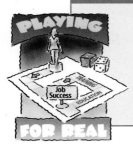

## Visualize It!

I'm Chantal. I used to have a real mental block when it came to the forearm bones. I just couldn't remember which is the radius and which is the ulna. Then, I figured out how I could use imagery to help me remember. I pictured myself taking a patient's radial pulse—the end of the radius is located right beneath that pulse! Now, when I have to know the forearm bones, I just picture taking a pulse. The image in my head helps me remember which bone is the radius.

### Think in Pictures

Imagery helps you link concrete objects with images, like a picture of a tree with the word *tree*. It also links abstract concepts with symbols, like a heart shape for *love*. As you study, draw pictures or symbols to illustrate important concepts. These visual cues will give your brain yet another way to remember the information.

### Use Color Coding

Colors can give meaning to the information you're studying as well. For example, you could use a variety of highlighters to color-code your lecture notes according to topic. You also could use color to indicate key points or to mark two or more related concepts in your textbook. Using color gives you a way to visually organize the material you're trying to learn and remember.

## Improve Your Efficiency of Studying

There are many ways to improve your efficiency as you study. Most of these techniques focus on helping you restate material in your own words. Here, we'll look at *reciprocal teaching* and *metalearning*.

### RECIPROCAL TEACHING

Reciprocal teaching is a method that will help you:

- summarize the content of a passage
- ask one good question about the main point of a passage
- clarify difficult parts of a passage
- predict what information will come in the next passage

Reciprocal teaching starts when you and the instructor read a short passage silently. Then the instructor summarizes, questions, clarifies, and predicts based on the passage. Next, you read another passage, but this time you do the summarizing, questioning, clarifying, and predicting. The instructor may give you clues, guidance, and other encouragement to help you master this method.

You can use the reciprocal teaching method in your individual study time after you've learned to use it. Read a passage or section, then summarize, question, clarify, and predict based on the passage. When you're done, you'll know the material inside and out.

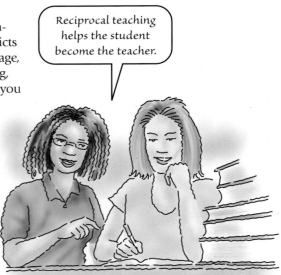

Reciprocal teaching helps the student become the teacher.

## METALEARNING

The prefix *meta-* means something that is aware of itself and refers to itself. Metalearning is a process where you ask yourself questions to become aware of your own motives, understanding, challenges, and goals.

In metalearning, you ask yourself a series of questions:

- *Why am I reading or listening to this?* In the metalearning process, you briefly state your purpose for studying certain material. Your purpose and goals set the stage for your study time.

- *What's the basic content of this material?* Preview material before you read. For long or complex material, translate your preview into a chapter map or outline. You also might want to write what you know about the topic and what you'd like to know or think you will know once you're done studying.

- *What are the orientation questions?* Orientation questions give background information on a topic or concept by asking about definitions, examples, types, relationships, or comparisons. The purpose of using orientation questions is to see how many questions you can ask about the material and how many answers you can find.

- *What's really important in this material?* Identify information you should focus on, ignore, or just skim. As in planning ahead, this helps you figure out where to spend your time. If you can't decide whether something is important or whether it should be skimmed or ignored, assume it's important.

- *How would I put this information in my own words?* Putting things in your own words is called paraphrasing. Paraphrasing helps you understand concepts better and identify gaps in your learning right away. Make sure you can put unique terminology for each subject into your own words.

- *How can I draw the information?* Visual learners can get a lot out of drawing the information they're studying. Representing information in pictures is very useful for building understanding.

- *How does the information fit with what I already know?* If you already have a solid foundation of knowledge about a topic, you can learn new things about that topic more easily.

## Rest, Relax, and Eat Right

As you study, your brain needs time to sort information and store it in your memory. To do that, your brain needs rest. Have you ever had a busy day at work and then dreamt about doing the same tasks? That's no accident. During deep sleep, the brain keeps right on sorting and storing information, saving important information, and forgetting unimportant details. By getting enough rest and relaxation, your brain can take a break from processing information, allowing it to catch up.

As Chapter 3 explains, what you eat also affects how your brain functions. A healthy, balanced diet gives you the energy and nutrition you need for studying.

## Reward Yourself

After studying, reward yourself for a successful study session. The reward can be something small, such as allowing yourself to watch a television show in the evening. What the reward itself isn't as important as getting a good feeling about the work you've done. And a positive attitude toward studying, as you learned earlier in this chapter, will motivate you to keep at it!

# STUDY GROUPS

Most of the study techniques we've been discussing so far in this chapter are things you can use on your own to learn and remember information, but they also work well when you study with others in a group. Study groups also allow for additional ways of learning and can be one of the best ways for students to master their course material.

Study groups may be informal, as simple as talking with a friend in the same class about an upcoming test of project due. More formal groups involving two or three others can be organized and scheduled for regular time. Both types of study groups can be very effective.

## Study Groups—Informal or Formal?

Being a part of a study group can help you learn and study course material. Even if your study group is not always able to answer your questions, teaching others can be a good way to learn. Explaining difficult concepts to someone else will help you review the information and get a firm grasp of important points. Going over course material with other students is an excellent way to help you understand it better and move it firmly into your long-term memory. This process can work in both informal and formal study groups.

### INFORMAL STUDY GROUPS

Students often get together before or after class to go over the material. These are informal groups where you are under no obligation to attend. When joining with others even in an informal group, however, you are expected to contribute to the discussion.

If you notice students gathering after class, hang around and see what they're talking about. If they're going over class material, introduce yourself and see if you can participate, too. Remember the discussion of networking in Chapter 4—studying with others is a great way also to build your network. Once you've discovered others in your class with whom you study well, consider making a more formal study group with them.

### FORMAL STUDY GROUPS

A formal study group is more organized. Students in the same class purposefully decide to get together to study, usually periodically during the school term. It usually helps to have a scheduled time to study together in a formal group rather than having to depend on casually finding someone in the class to talk with.

Review the section in Chapter 4 on networking with other students for suggestions on how to form a formal study group.

## Building a Study Group

A formal study group doesn't just happen—you and other students have to put in a little effort to get it started and keep it on track. You'll need to consider a few issues to build an effective group:

- How many students in the group?
- How and when to schedule meetings?
- Where to meet?
- How to ensure everyone participates fairly?

## IF THREE'S A CROWD . . .

It's easier to stay on task when everyone in the group is interested in the same thing—studying. If the group becomes too large (more than four or five members), it can be broken down into smaller groups. Meeting with a smaller number of people makes it easier to review all the necessary material and answer each other's questions.

## SCHEDULING MEETINGS BY THE BOOK

It's great to have a regularly scheduled time for a study group—a time when everyone comes prepared to discuss a certain topic. Meeting regularly to go over material helps you all come up with new ideas and approaches.

> When participating in an online discussion, only talk to people you know and trust.

It can be hard to find a time when busy people can meet. Do the best you can to come up with a regular meeting time, such as every week or every 2 weeks. If evenings are best, go with that. If two half-hour meetings a week are better for everyone's schedule than one hour-long meeting per week, go with two half-hour meetings.

### When You Can't Find a Scheduling Solution

If you are unable to find a time to meet in person, you create an online group site or message board. Everyone can visit the group site and contribute to it whenever they're free. You can create a group on websites like Yahoo Groups where members log in and talk via instant message boards. But be vigilant about keeping passwords strictly within the network, for safety's sake. You'll want to avoid having strangers posting on your site.

### Where to Meet

There are many places for a study group to meet. Finding the one that is right for you can take a little trial and error—what seems perfect at first may not actually work out later. Keep at it until you get to the right place.

Many students find it easiest to meet on campus in a common area or in a library discussion room (just make sure you're not out in the middle of the library disrupting others). If your regular meeting time falls during the school day, this may be the best option for you.

Meeting off campus may work better if your meeting time falls after classes have ended for the day. It also may work better for members who are not on campus (professionals in the workplace or students at another campus). In this case, meet at a centrally located coffee shop or take turns hosting the group at your homes.

Just remember—safety first! Make sure you know everyone in your group well before you agree to meet them somewhere or invite them to your home.

## Keeping the Group Focused

When it comes to study groups, remember the four Cs. A successful study group will have members who are:

- committed—interested in learning the material
- contributors—willing to share their knowledge
- compatible—able to overlook differences and focus on studying together
- considerate—willing to arrive at meetings on time

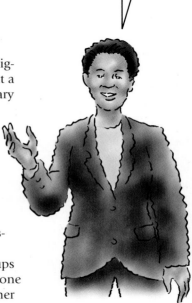

*When forming a study group, remember the four Cs. All group members should be Committed Contributors who are Compatible and Considerate.*

To have productive meetings, your group might choose to designate a "timekeeper." This person keeps everyone moving along at a good pace. That way, your group will be sure to cover the necessary material during each session.

You might also need to designate a "gatekeeper." This person makes sure the group stays focused on appropriate topics. When people start to discuss things unrelated to the course material, that person can remind everyone to stay focused.

It's everyone's responsibility to prepare before meeting with the group. You should be familiar with the material you'll be studying together, even if you have questions about it. Your questions may be helpful to the rest of the group. Make sure you can explain other concepts in your own words. Successful study groups have a give-and-take. If the group answers your questions about one concept, you may be able to return the favor by explaining another idea to the rest of the group.

## Giving Your Two Cents

Students in an effective study group listen to every member because every member has something valuable to say. Even though not everyone is an expert or has 20 years' experience, all students should be studying hard, make the most of what they do know, and want to learn more.

In an effective study group, all members share their ideas and information. No one should be worried that what they say will be taken out of context or used to try to gain an unfair advantage. No one tries to gain from other people's experience without sharing their own. In a good group, everyone contributes fairly and benefits equally.

## THE HUDDLE

A study group should be made up of people you like and respect. A study session should be stress-free and it's OK if it sometimes includes informal conversation. You should be able to laugh, share funny stories, and confide your doubts and worries without being concerned that the whole school will find out about it later.

For example, a football player wouldn't leave the huddle and then tell the other team what the next play is going to be. That would be disloyal to teammates. Be sure to have the same respect for the other members of your network. If someone mentions any personal matter in the group, avoid the urge to gossip. Keep personal information private.

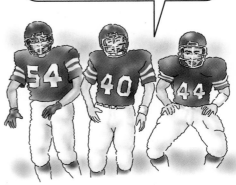

*Teammates trust each other—be the kind of person your study group can trust. If another member mentions something in confidence, avoid the urge to gossip.*

# MORE RESOURCES FOR STUDYING

We've been looking at how you and your study group can use your textbook, class notes, and materials from your instructor when studying. In addition to all this, there's another whole world of supplemental materials out there to help you learn. Never discount the value of using additional materials when studying, even when not assigned or required by the instructor.

## Using Supplemental Materials

Using supplemental material is another way to accommodate your personal learning style. If you have a hard time learning information from a lecture or a textbook, it's especially helpful to supplement your education. When the same information is presented to you in a variety of ways, you'll learn more and have better recall of important points. You may also use supplemental material as a way of finding out more about an interesting topic covered in one of your classes. Whatever your reason may be, making use of supplemental material gives you an advantage as a student.

Your textbook may include a toll-free phone number that you can call for help with finding supplemental materials. Browse the text materials near the front of the book for information about resources available for students.

### TEXTBOOK CDS

Textbooks often come with CDs or workbooks that are loaded with practice quizzes, sample test questions, games, and other learning tools designed to increase learning. Often, these involve the same information as the textbook but in a different format. For example, some CDs may include interactive exercises. This can be helpful to students who have a difficult time understanding the material as it's presented in the textbook. CDs also can be helpful to students looking for ways to improve their recall of information in the textbook.

## SOFTWARE AND ONLINE RESOURCES

There are many different kinds of educational software that you may find helpful. Such software may be available on a student disk with a textbook, at a computer lab at your school or library, online, or elsewhere. Types of software that are particularly beneficial to students include:

- practice exercises
- tutorials
- simulations
- assessments
- video and audio podcasts

Software such as this may be included on a CD or DVD accompanying your textbook. Some commercially available software may also be helpful, depending on your particular field of study. Finally, the same sorts of materials are often available at websites—like the student resources on this book's companion website! Aside from requiring an Internet connection, supplementary material on the Web is often, in practical terms, indistinguishable from software running on your own computer.

### Practice Makes Perfect

Some website software provides practice exercises. These may be in the form of quizzes you can take or problems you can solve. Their purpose is to help students learn and remember facts and vocabulary. They can also aid in your understanding of how different concepts are related. The more you practice, the more you'll be required to use your new knowledge. This increases your ability to remember and comprehend the material in your textbook.

Students with full-time jobs or families may prefer to use tutorial software instead of taking extra time to meet with a tutor.

### Your Own Private Tutor

If you find yourself lost even after attending lectures and getting clarification from your instructor, tutorial software or websites can help. These are designed to teach concepts. Although they may include brief quizzes to assess your level of knowledge, the main focus is instruction. The material may be presented in several different formats, making use of text, images, audio, and video. They may also be interactive, with content covered depending on student responses.

## Is This for Real?

Simulations are another type of educational software or Web application. Simulations are computerized versions of real-life experiences. They are interactive and often require decision making on the part of the student. Health profession students can use these programs to learn or hone their clinical skills. The beauty of simulations is that they are forgiving of mistakes made during the learning process. After all, it's better to make a mistake while caring for a simulated patient than to make one while caring for an actual patient!

## How Am I Doing?

Assessment software and websites can be beneficial to students and instructors alike. On one hand, computerized testing helps students determine their level of knowledge. As a student, being aware of how much you know can help you set goals for yourself. It allows you to focus on what you have yet to learn. On the other hand, assessments can also be helpful to instructors. Once they are able to determine their students' progress, they can adjust the curriculum appropriately.

## Podcasts

Instructors at some schools video or audio tape their lectures and make these available for students as podcasts that can be played on a computer or an mp3/mp4 device. If your school produces podcasts, your instructor will tell you about this. Because a recording cannot capture the full experience of attending class, don't consider a podcast a replacement for attending class—but it can be a helpful review when needed.

In addition, educational podcasts are available online or through "iTunes U." You do not need an iPod to view these videos or listen to audios; programs on many subjects are available to everyone through the free iTunes program or the websites of individual schools. For example, if you are having difficulty understanding the anatomy of a particular organ or body system, dozens of video podcasts are available to help walk you through this information. Podcasts from other schools do not replace your textbook, of course, and may contain more or less detail than you need to understand for your course, but when used as supplementary material, they can enrich your understanding.

## The Wonderful World Wide Web

As described in Chapter 7, you can find a wealth of supplemental material online for any course you're taking. Just remember to stay safe when on the Internet.

- Make sure websites are trustworthy. Websites that end in .gov or .edu generally contain reliable information.
- Make sure any website you use is accurate (up-to-date and unbiased). Personal websites, like blogs, may have a lot of information, but there is no guarantee that the information is accurate.
- Only use websites that are free. And never give out your own personal information to use a website.
- If possible, get a list of reliable websites from your instructor.
- Textbook publishers also often have websites where you can find lots of resources to help you study.

## STUDY SKILLS FOR MATH AND SCIENCE

Many people have something we call "math anxiety" or feel apprehensive about taking science courses. Perhaps the world of numbers or science seems strange and alien to them. Or maybe they had a bad experience with a math or science class when they were younger. It can be hard to overcome this anxiety, especially in a society where this anxiety is accepted as normal and understandable.

But overcoming this anxiety is important. Math is used in daily life and math classes are unavoidable when you're in school. Most health care careers also require some familiarity with the sciences, particularly those involving the human body. You'll want to be able to approach these classes with confidence and a fresh attitude. You may need to pay special attention to math and science, then, in your studies.

## Why Is Math So Important?

Many people struggle through high school math, hoping or assuming they'll never need to deal with it later in life. But math is all around you. Health care professionals need to be competent in math to perform many tasks:

- measuring solutions
- figuring dosages
- converting pounds to kilograms for weights

- creating department budgets
- scheduling staff assignments
- handling patients' claims and bills

## Math Myths

One of the reasons it's hard to overcome math anxiety is that people believe things about math that just aren't true. Let's look at some of the most common math myths and how to shake them.

### "I'M JUST NOT GOOD AT MATH"

People think of math as much harder than other topics, a kind of mystery where numbers are a foreign language. Sometimes, students are told they just can't do math and should leave it alone.

Are you a problem-solver? Are you driven to succeed? If your answer is yes, then you probably have greater math aptitude than you think. Math is all about solving problems. All you have to learn is the language of math—numbers—and you can start solving math problems.

### "MY CALCULATOR DOES THE MATH FOR ME"

A calculator is just a tool to do math problems faster. A calculator might be able to multiply more easily than you can. But it can't tell you what the $x$ stands for in an algebra equation or why an $x$ is used in that problem in the first place. It can't explain what a square root is or how it's used in real life.

Think of your calculator as a tool to help you perform basics like addition, subtraction, multiplication, and division faster and with fewer errors. But be sure to learn how math really works. Your calculator can only take you so far.

### "I DON'T USE MATH IN MY LIFE—WHY LEARN IT?"

In fact, math is used in everyday life, even though you may not always see it or realize it. For instance, learning how to make conversions between different systems of measurement will help you calculate proper medication dosages for patients. Learning about other math concepts will allow you to create budgets at work and at home and complete many other vital tasks. Basic math is needed to balance your checkbook, understand a mortgage payment or interest on a car loan, and cope with many day-to-day aspects of life.

## Success in Math Class

Some students dread math class. Somehow, they have the feeling they're supposed to know the material already. They're embarrassed to admit they don't understand a problem or a concept. But a math

> No matter where you go in your health career, you'll need good math skills. Take the time to hone them now!

class is where you *learn math*. If there's any place in the world where you can put your math fears on the table and conquer them, it's math class. Here are some resources to use that will make math class a success for you.

> *A math tutor can give you the encouragement you need to keep working at it!*

## TALK TO YOUR INSTRUCTOR

Many students are embarrassed to tell their instructor they don't understand something. But your instructor is there to help you. If you hide the fact that you don't understand something, your instructor can't help you. But if you let your instructor know, you can get the help you need.

## USE YOUR TEXTBOOK

Most math textbooks have plenty of practice questions, either at the end of each chapter or grouped together in the back of the book. Use these practice questions. Working through them helps you see some of the underlying patterns of a concept or technique and helps get you in the swing of using certain functions or solutions. Never skip over math questions or problems, because it's likely the next material you'll need to understand will build on what you're reading and doing now. If you skip over something that doesn't seem clear, the problem will only grow worse.

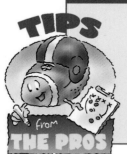

## Personal Trainer

**TIPS from THE PROS**

There are people other than your instructor who can help you with math. You can find mentors at school or in your own family. And tutors are usually available—just ask your instructor or the secretary in the math department. Check bulletin boards in the math department and student centers, too; you'll probably find many ads posted that offer tutoring services. Some may even be free. There are also interactive online tutoring sites. Finally, a math study group can be a huge help. So get off the bench and get some help tackling your toughest math problems!

## WRITE IT ALL DOWN

Do each step of a math problem on paper, not in your head. Even if you know the formula well, write down each step. It helps you focus and gets your mind in the problem-solving groove. Just like a great musician still practices scales each day, you should write down even basic steps. It can also help you find careless errors in your work.

## READ CAREFULLY

Get in the habit of reading very carefully when you go through a math problem. Most errors occur when you misread a problem. Read through each problem out loud so that each part of it makes sense to you. Sometimes, you might think you see "add" when the symbol actually says "divide"; talking through the problem helps eliminate these kinds of errors.

## SEE WHAT'S NOT THERE

If you don't understand the solution to a problem, there might be something missing from the problem itself. People do make mistakes! Prepare a list of problems you are unable to work out and discuss each one with your instructor. This way, you'll learn to see what you're missing.

## DO THE MATH!

Students sometimes think that the assigned materials are the only ones they should use. But supplementary materials can give you fresh examples and practice problems. It's worth it to get these extra materials. Before you invest in one, make sure it has a lot of examples and step-by-step instructions. It should include proofs or derivations for the formulas it uses. Remember, different authors might use different notation systems, so be sure to familiarize yourself with them.

# Preparing for Math Class

Math is sequential—every concept builds on a previous concept. If you miss one step, the next one won't make sense to you. That's why it's important to go to every class and set aside time each day to go over what you've learned. Here are the basics to review daily:

- vocabulary
- basic formulas
- working cooperatively
- testing yourself

## TALK THE TALK

Like many subjects, math has a specialized vocabulary. If you don't know the most common math terms, you'll have trouble with problems you could otherwise solve. Make a list of key words and study them. This list can include words emphasized by your instructor or your textbook, as well as words you find you have trouble remembering.

Treat math like a foreign language; you learn a language by picking out vocabulary words and memorizing them. You have to know how to pronounce vocabulary words, what they mean, and when they are used.

## KNOW THE FORMULAS

Like vocabulary, math formulas form the basis for solving math problems. It's valuable to understand why a formula works the way it does. It's especially important to memorize basic formulas, as these are the formulas you'll use most often.

## TEAMWORK

Usually, math isn't taught collaboratively. Students are rarely broken into groups to work something out. That's one of the reasons many students fear math: they are on their own, left to sink or swim.

But many instructors have come to realize the benefits of letting students work with a partner. Once you find a good partner, you can help each other solve problems. A partner can bring you:

- *Another point of view.* This helps you see more possibilities, thus improving your learning.

- *Increased personal accountability.* If someone is depending on you to help them study and learn, you will take that responsibility seriously.

- *An audience.* If you can explain a concept to your partner, you can explain it to the instructor on a test.

- *Praise and encouragement.* You and your partner will root for each other and provide positive feedback, helping create confidence.

Even if your instructor does not pair you with a partner, remember that you can set up your own study group to go over the math you're learning in class. Often, it's easiest to learn how to apply formulas when talking them through with other students. Just make sure you really understand it! If you let others do your thinking for you, you'll have trouble with future math problems that build on the understanding of these formulas.

Working as a team can help you tackle the toughest math problems.

# Studying Science

Much of the preceding discussion of math and studying math is also true of the sciences and studying science. In fact, many people have the same anxiety or apprehensions about science as they do about math, and understanding many of the sciences requires understanding mathematical formulas.

Try to apply all the same principles when studying for your science courses. Most important, don't be afraid to ask your instructor questions.

If you feel frustrated reading scientific information or texts, take a moment and remind yourself that health care is largely based on science. To understand how illness can be prevented or treated, we need to understand how the body works, beginning with basic biology. To understand how to take x-ray exposures and process images, we need to understand the basic physics of x-ray beams and their interaction with matter. Even to understand medical terminology, we need to feel comfortable with scientific language. Although you may not immediately see the value of something scientific you are studying, rest assured that later on, as you enter your chosen health care career, that knowledge will have a big payoff because you better understand the reasons for actions you take on the job. The more you understand of the scientific side of health care, the more deeply involved you'll feel in your work—and the happier you'll be with your career choice.

## CHAPTER SUMMARY

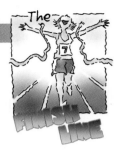

- Set goals for each study session to give yourself a game plan to follow and to make the most efficient use of your study time.

- Get organized. Organize your school papers (notes, syllabi, schedule, etc.) for quick and easy access.

- Consider a space's lighting, temperature, and surroundings when choosing a study space.

- Get more out of studying by using strategies to improve your concentration and memory.

- Use different study methods, such as repeating information, taking short breaks, and using acronyms or acrostics.

- Rest, exercise, and proper nutrition will give you the energy you need to stay alert and focused as you study.

- Develop good study groups that will help you learn and support your academic goals.

- Use supplemental material to increase your learning. Resources, such as textbook CDs, educational software, the Internet, and online instruction, can provide benefits beyond the classroom.

## REVIEW QUESTIONS

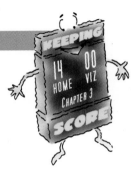

1. What are at least two tips for getting organized?

2. Name at least three different study strategies.

3. What are four characteristics that members of a successful study group should have? (Hint: Remember the four Cs.)

4. How does assessment software benefit students and instructors?

5. Explain why it's not a good idea to expect a calculator to do all of your math for you.

## CHAPTER ACTIVITIES

1. Study Space Checklist: Review *Scope out a Study Area* and make a list of the characteristics you find most important for a study space. Then locate at least two places that meet your criteria—your principal study area and a backup when the first is not available for any reason.

2. Getting Organized Checklist: Review *Getting Organized* and compose a checklist of things to do in order to organize your paperwork for each class.

3. Study Group Planning: Choose one of your classes and look around at the other students in the room. Based on what you have observed about them from how they interact in the classroom, select three students you'd ideally like to have in your study group. (If you haven't already formed a group for that class, talk to these students soon to see if they're interested.)

## CHAPTER 9

# Test-Taking Skills

*On completion of this chapter and the learning activities you will be able to:*

- Understand and fight test anxiety

- Prepare and study for tests

- Use different strategies to do well on objective, subjective, and other tests

- Succeed on math tests

- Know how to calculate grades

- Prepare for a certification or licensure exam

Does anyone you know *love* taking tests? Probably not! Tests are something all students face and tests cause almost everyone anxiety. In this chapter, you'll find out how to plan and prepare for tests so you can improve your test-taking abilities and feel more confident. You'll also learn about special skills for managing test anxiety. Tips and guidelines will be presented for math tests and special exams such as those required for certification or licensure in many health care careers.

## HEALTH AND STRESS MANAGEMENT

Doing well on a test starts long before you take out your pencil on the big day. It starts with how well you take care of your mind and your body. Yes, studying is certainly key to your success, but how you care for your health and how you manage stress are very important, too.

Here's a quick review of what Chapter 3 describes about caring for your body for maximum functioning and low stress.

- Regular exercise can lower stress, keep you fit and looking good, and make you feel better mentally and physically.

- Sometimes rest is more important than completing every task on your daily to-do list.

- A balanced and nutritious diet is important for your health and managing stress.

- Breathing and relaxation techniques or yoga can help release tension.

Chapter 3 also explains that your mind needs recharging. Here's a review of some of the techniques you can use:

- *Keep negative thoughts under control.* Use positive imagery to move your mind toward your goals and away from your fears.

- *Calm your body to calm your mind.* When you have negative thoughts, use body-calming techniques (such as those discussed in Chapter 3) to enter a more calm and relaxed state of mind.

- *Visualize yourself achieving your goals and overcoming obstacles.* Think about how you feel when you visualize these things and remember that feeling when negativity rears its head.

- *Build a social support network.* Family, friends, classmates, coworkers, and people who share your interests are all good choices for a social support network. They give you an outlet for discussing your problems with people who care for you and want to help.

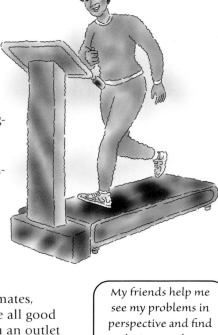

> Running makes me feel tired right now, but later it will give me the energy I need!

> My friends help me see my problems in perspective and find solutions to them.

## TEST ANXIETY

Remember what *eustress* means? That's right—good healthy, levels of stress. But most of us are more familiar with *distress*—high, unhealthy levels of stress. Most students experience some stress at test time, but for some, increased stress at test time interferes with their ability to think. They know the material. They've studied hard and effectively. But they just get so tense at test time that they can't put down the right answers. The way to beat test anxiety is to first recognize it and then prepare to fight it!

## Are You an Anxious Student?

Part of recognizing test anxiety is figuring out whether you're an anxious student. The following sections describe several different characteristics of anxious students.

### FEELINGS, TOO MANY FEELINGS . . .

Really anxious students go back and forth between focusing on new material and thinking about how nervous they are. They find it difficult to maintain their concentration during a lecture or a reading session. They keep noticing their discomfort and think, "I'm so tense—I just can't do this!" Because very anxious students' attention is focused on worrying about doing a bad job, being criticized, or feeling embarrassed, they may miss the information they need to learn.

### LOST IN THE DETAILS

Anxious students often have poor study habits. It's hard for them to learn if the material is:

- disorganized
- broken down in many parts
- difficult to understand
- focused on memorization

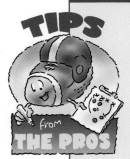

### Avoid the Big Freeze-Up

The most common test anxiety experience is a mental block or "freeze-up." Although many students experience some level of this, students with severe test anxiety might read a test question over and over and never take in its meaning. Other symptoms of severe mental block include:

- doing poorly on a test after proving you know the material during class and in study groups
- feeling sweaty, shaky, or physically ill before and during a test
- obsessing over how well you're doing compared with other students
- thinking about how to get out of finishing the test, such as by faking an illness

If you're so overwhelmed with test anxiety that you can't do well on tests—even when you've attended every class, studied hard, and proven that you know the material—talk to your instructor about it. Your instructor might have another solution you haven't thought of. Alternately, ask a peer tutor or friend to "test" you with questions you haven't seen and a set time limit for completing the work. Taking practice tests beforehand can help you ease into the real thing.

In these situations, anxious students are very easily distracted by irrelevant or minor details of the tasks at hand. They can't see the forest for the trees, which means they focus on details and miss the main point.

## Recognize Test Anxiety

You've read about what goes wrong for very anxious students. But a little anxiety can be a good thing. Slight anxiety can improve your focus and mental sharpness. It keeps you from feeling complacent and helps you stay motivated to study. But if you consistently feel nervous and distracted, test anxiety is probably taking over.

Test anxiety may produce many effects before and during a test. Here are some common effects of test anxiety:

- freezing up, when your brain doesn't take in the meaning of questions or you have to read questions over and over to understand them
- panicking about tough questions or about time running out before you're done
- worrying about the grade you'll receive
- becoming easily distracted, daydreaming, or thinking about how you could escape taking the test
- feeling nervous about your ability to do well or about how you'll do compared to others
- having physical symptoms of stress, such as sweating, nausea, muscle tension, and headaches
- feeling like you're not interested in the topic or like you don't care how well you do on the test

## Prepare to Fight Anxiety

The key to staying on top of anxiety for most successful students is using a combination of techniques to prepare for tests. This section discusses tips and guidelines all students can use. Remember that you need to prepare your mind and body. Keeping this balance will help you overcome your test anxiety and do your best.

### STUDY WELL

Studying well is the best preparation for a test—and the best cure for test anxiety. Studying can give you a sense of accomplishment that boosts your self-confidence. When you know the material backward and forward, you won't feel as nervous going into the test.

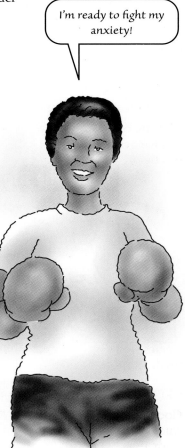

*I'm ready to fight my anxiety!*

## RELAX YOUR MIND

Relaxation, along with other stress-reduction techniques, can help lessen test anxiety. When your body is relaxed, your mind is free to absorb new information. Try using breathing exercises or meditation to clear your mind.

## THINK POSITIVELY

Test anxiety can result from low self-esteem. Focus on being positive about tests. Say to yourself, "I've studied hard and I know this material. I can do this!" Being prepared and having a positive attitude often lead to success.

## GIVE YOURSELF A BREAK

If you start to feel anxious during a test, consider doing something to break the tension, such as putting down your pencil, closing your eyes, and taking a few slow deep breaths. If your shoulders are hunched, make a conscious effort to lower them and relax. If the instructor allows, you might even get up and sharpen your pencil or ask a question. Sometimes you can feel anxiety because you're physically tired and need a break.

## GET YOUR ZZZs

Rest and relaxation are great fatigue-fighters. You can do more when you feel rested and relaxed than when you're tired. Try using these tips before your next test.

- Get enough sleep—at least 7 to 8 hours at a time.
- Change activities from time to time.
- Exercise on a regular basis.
- Relax by allowing yourself breaks for TV, music, friends, or light reading.

## SIT UP STRAIGHT

Your posture matters when you're studying or taking a test. If you're sitting in an uncomfortable position, it stresses your muscles. This stress is communicated to your brain, which in turn creates anxiety. Slouching can hurt your back and make you feel tired. Sit up straight and allow your concentration to return.

## EAT WELL, TEST WELL

Good nutrition keeps you healthy. It also can improve your study habits and test-taking skills. Class time, work time, and study time often conflict with meal times. To counter this, avoid skipping meals and eat nutritious snacks between sessions.

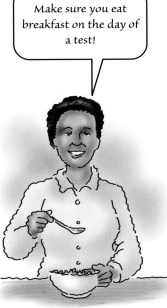

Make sure you eat breakfast on the day of a test!

## If You Get Sick . . .

Even the healthiest person can get sick. When you're ill, you can't perform well on a test. So, if you feel very ill as a test approaches, contact the instructor. This shows you care about your performance and about missing the test. You may be able to work out an arrangement with the instructor and this will help you avoid anxiety about

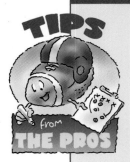

## Defeat Test Anxiety!

Here's a checklist of things to do the next time you're feeling nervous about a test.

Before the test:

- Talk to your instructor and classmates about what the test will cover.
- Use the study skills you learned in Chapter 8. Develop a method that works for you!
- Divide your study time over several days instead of trying to review everything the night before the test. Use the time management skills you learned in Chapter 2.
- When studying, use all your resources, including your textbook, lecture notes, and completed homework assignments.
- Create 3 × 5 cards for all key concepts or formulas that might appear on the test. Use the flash cards to practice and test your memory.
- Take a practice test. Find a room that's free of distractions and give yourself a specific amount of time to complete the test.
- Try to avoid studying right before taking the test. Put those notes away and take some time to relax!
- Arrive 5 minutes early so you'll be ready when the instructor begins the test. Just don't arrive too early—sitting in an empty classroom or listening to other students' nervous chattering might make you feel anxious.

During the test:

- Break the tension. If your instructor allows it, get up to ask a question, sharpen your pencil, or get a drink.
- Focus on tensing and relaxing muscles in different parts of your body, such as your neck and shoulders. Then close your eyes and take a few deep breaths.
- Calm your nerves by putting the test into perspective. Life will go on after the test is over. Remember that doing your best is sufficient.
- Think of something calm and soothing when you feel test anxiety is getting the best of you.

postponing the test. Be sure to follow all your doctor's instructions so you can get well as soon as possible. Avoid using sick time as study time and get the rest you need.

## Stay on Schedule

When a test approaches, keep things as normal as possible. If you normally take a walk before dinner, keep up with your routine instead of skipping your walk to study. If you usually sleep 8 hours a night, avoid the urge to cram until 2:00 AM. Breaking good habits will only contribute to your mental and physical stress.

# PREPARING AND PLANNING AHEAD

When it comes to test taking, preparation is important. Knowing *what* you need to do *before* you have to do it gives you time to work out the best *way* to do it.

## Know What Will Be Covered

You can't study well for a test if you don't know what kind of test it will be. If you know what kind of test to expect, you can put your study time to good use. Objective tests, such as short answer, sentence completion, multiple choice, matching, and true/false, require you to remember facts and details and to recognize related material. Essay and oral tests require you to make good arguments about general topics and to support your arguments with critical details.

### SIZE IT UP

You should always attend class, but it's especially important leading up to a test. Your instructor will probably explain the format of the test during class time. If not, visit your instructor during office hours and ask these questions:

- Will the test be comprehensive or will it cover select material only (like a few chapters)?
- Approximately how many questions will there be?
- How will the questions be weighted? For example, will multiple choice questions be worth 5 points each, whereas essays will be worth 20 points?
- How much will this test count toward my final grade?
- What materials will I need? A calculator? Scrap paper?

## LEARN FROM THE PAST

If you've already taken tests in the course or attended another course given by the same instructor, you probably have some idea of what the upcoming test will be like. For example, you might know that the instructor focuses on details rather than principles or that sometimes uses trick questions.

But if it's your first test for a particular course or instructor, you can still do a little extra preparation. Ask your instructor if practice tests or exams from the past are available for students to study. But remember, although past tests can give you an idea of what the test may be like, you won't see the same questions on your upcoming test.

## LEARN FROM THE CLASS

Think about how you've learned things in class so far. Which topics has the instructor spent the most time discussing? Have you focused on details or large concepts in class discussions? Some instructors offer review sessions before the test. If your instructor does this, be there and be prepared. Plan ahead of time for the review session by writing down the questions you'd like to ask.

# Get Ready, Get Set. . .

Give yourself a head start before you begin studying for an upcoming test. Thorough preparation short-circuits anxiety. The class schedule likely lists test dates and other deadlines. Put those test dates in your planning calendar. If your instructor didn't provide a class schedule at the beginning of the term, ask about approximate dates of tests.

## CREATE A GAME PLAN

First, create an organized study plan. For example, you could set aside some time to study each day for a week before the test. Studying every day keeps the material fresh in your mind. Give yourself enough time to review your lecture notes, study materials, and old tests (if possible) several times. Choose a good place to study. Consider your study group; you can ask each other questions of the sort likely to appear on the test. Commit to studying and you'll be as prepared as possible for the test.

You might already review your notes after each class, which is good practice. But remember that it's not enough before a test. You'll need more intense review. In some classes, you may even have unannounced pop quizzes before a test. In those cases, you'll be glad you spent extra time studying!

## The Trouble with Cramming

The trouble with cramming is that it doesn't work. You simply can't cram data into the brain and have it stick. Most of the information disappears in a few hours. And, by the time you're sitting down to the test, your brain is so tired that it can't retrieve most of the data it did manage to retain. As a result, you "blank out" and are unable to answer questions you might otherwise have easily answered.

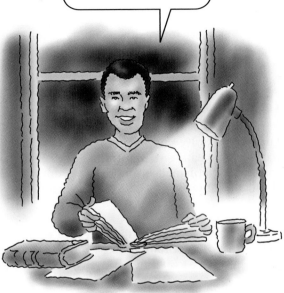

*I can't cram in any more information—my brain is too full of fatigue!*

## Trying to Beat the Clock

When you have a test coming up and you feel unprepared for it, the best thing to do is stay calm and focused. Double-check with your instructor or a classmate about the format of the test. Use your textbook to create a master study outline. Focus on chapter headings, summaries, highlighted words, formulas, definitions, and the first and last sentences of every paragraph. Write key points and an outline of each chapter on notebook paper.

When you're done outlining in this way, review your class notes and handouts. Make some "must-know" flash cards for what you feel is the most important information. Flip through the flash cards until you're too tired to continue. Make sure to wake up at least 1 hour before the test to review your outline and flip through the flash cards again.

## BRING THE RIGHT EQUIPMENT

Remember to bring the right "equipment" to your study session. A student trying to study without a textbook is like a football player showing up to practice without a helmet! So, before you begin studying, gather all your review materials, textbooks, and notes. Look for information about the main terms, facts, concepts, themes, problems, questions, and issues that were covered in those materials. It's especially handy to compare the way your textbook covers an idea or concept with how your instructor covered it in class.

When you're studying for a test, it's not a good use of time to try to reread entire chapters of your textbook. Instead, armed with your knowledge about what kinds of questions will be asked and which topics will be covered, use your textbook's index and glossary to look up just those topics. Find definitions of key terms in the glossary and look for important details in handouts and other supplementary material. Make lists of definitions and rehearse them.

## MAKE A STUDY SHEET

Summarize your notes on one piece of paper. Review this study sheet, then place it face down and try to re-create your notes from memory. Think about where each topic was placed on the page. That way, when you encounter a certain topic on the test, you can flash back to your notes page and actually "see" the information.

### Equations and Graphs

For math or science tests, practice your skills by rewriting equations and graphs. Solve sample problems and write out formulas. If you have trouble with certain formulas or graphs, make a separate sheet for those troublemakers and review it during gaps in your schedule throughout the day.

### Main Terms

For short-answer tests, go through your textbook or lecture notes and make a list of important terms. Then add the definitions and think of an example of each term that you could use in a short answer.

### Practice Run

For an essay test, prepare by doing a practice run. First, look at previous assignments and tests to see how essay questions are worded. Then, choose a topic from the material you're studying now and develop an essay question. Finally, write an answer for your essay question, giving yourself as much time as you'll have during your upcoming test. (See *Subjective Tests* for tips on how to develop a good essay.)

## My Study Strategy

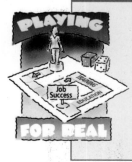

My name is Sujala. I'm studying to become a pharmacy technician. When I have a big test coming up, I do a couple of things to prepare. First, I talk with the instructor and find out what kinds of questions the test will have—multiple choice, short answer, or other kinds. Then I go through my notes and make practice questions out of them. For instance, I put my notes into multiple choice format. That way, I can see how the information looks in test form. I make up a study sheet, too. The night before the test, I get a babysitter to watch my kids so I can review the study sheet and get it down pat.

## BE YOUR OWN COACH

Giving yourself a practice test allows you to be your own coach. Practice tests help you recognize the topics you struggle with most, which focuses your studying. To make a practice test, look at your study sheet and turn it into a series of questions. Then, answer the questions as if you are really taking a test. Sit in a quiet room and give yourself a certain amount of time to work. You may feel less anxiety when you take the real test if it feels familiar.

After you complete the practice test, use your study resources to check your answers. Spend extra time studying the questions you answered incorrectly.

> Be your own coach when it comes to studying! Give yourself a practice test to figure out how well you know the material.

## GAME DAY

On the day of the test, there are several things you can do to make sure you're in top condition.

- *Rest.* You need at least 7 to 8 hours of sleep the night before a test.
- *Eat small meals.* Breakfast is the most important. Just avoid eating too much or you'll feel sleepy.
- *Avoid caffeine.* You don't want to be jittery.
- *Exercise.* Even a short exercise session will help you feel mentally and physically invigorated.
- *Have your test materials ready to go.* Do this the night before so you won't waste time frantically searching for something on test day. Include all written materials, notes, pens, erasers, pencils, calculators, and whatever else is allowed or required.
- *Arrive on time.* Make sure you wear a watch. Not only will this help you avoid being late or having to rush to be on time, but during the test you can track how much time is left. It's best to arrive 5 minutes early so you can be seated and ready by the time the test begins.
- *Pay attention to the test instructions.* Do this before you rush right to the questions. Read or listen to directions, such as "copy the question" or "show your work." Then, skim the test. Jot a few notes that bring bits of information to mind. By reviewing questions quickly in advance, your brain can work on answers to longer questions while you complete shorter questions.
- *Budget test time efficiently.* After you skim the test, think about how to budget your time. Think about how much time you have to finish the test, the total number of questions, the type and difficulty of each question, and the point value of each. If you start to lag during the test, don't stress. You can rebound by adjusting your schedule.

# TEST-TAKING STRATEGIES

You'll take many different kinds of tests during your student career, each of which requires unique strategies. There are objective tests, such as multiple choice and true/false, and subjective tests, such as essays. There are vocabulary, reading comprehension, open-book, take-home, oral, and standardized tests as well.

You've probably seen some of these test types before. You might even have an idea of which kinds of tests you find easier or more difficult. But no matter where your strengths or weaknesses lie, all students can use the same basic tips to improve their test-taking skills. And once you can conquer any test, you'll be well on your way to success!

## Bloom's Taxonomy and Question Types

Before we look at different types of test questions commonly used, it's helpful to understand how instructors think about tests—and what it is they're actually testing. The system developed by Benjamin Bloom to explain different cognitive levels or ways of thinking has shaped how many educators think about what and how they want their students to learn. This is called Bloom's Taxonomy of the Cognitive Domain or sometimes Bloom's learning levels. The six learning levels are described in Chapter 5:

- knowledge
- comprehension
- application
- analysis
- synthesis
- evaluation

As you prepare for a test in any course, it helps to think also about these levels. Your primary consideration involves what learning activities your course focuses on and what kinds of test questions may be used to assess your mastery of that learning.

For example, let's say you have been learning how to take patients' vital signs—to take a temperature, measure blood pressure, and so on. Your instructor has emphasized that accuracy is the most important aspect of performing these skills. You need to perform each step in each procedure correctly. As described in Chapter 5, this learning is primarily in the first two levels of Bloom's Taxonomy: knowledge and comprehension. You have to remember exactly what steps to use, for example, in using blood pressure equipment. You also need to understand what you are doing—the comprehension level—in order to do your job well. You can expect, therefore, that a test that includes this topic will likely include knowledge and comprehension types of questions. As noted in Chapter 5, this means not only recalling pertinent information and facts but also being able to describe in your own words information such as how to take a blood pressure.

Although knowledge and comprehension may be most important for this learning, the next level in the taxonomy is likely also important: application. That is so because as you learned the steps for how to take a blood pressure, you also learned you may need to vary the equipment or process in different situations. Can you explain *why* to use a different blood pressure cuff for a child or an adult with a large arm—and how the readings you obtain may be inaccurate if you do not? Because the application learning level is also important for this topic, it's likely the test may include questions such as this also.

Remember that the three highest learning levels—analysis, synthesis, and evaluation—are involved in critical thinking. In these levels, it's not enough just to remember how to do something, why, and how to apply it in a new situation. Instead, you're expected to think more deeply about the issues involved. For example, you take a patient's temperature and find it normal, but an hour later, it is 3° F higher. Do you evaluate that fact as meaningful? Do you just record the information as you've been taught to and go on about your work, or do you decide this is a significant change you should report immediately to a physician or nurse in case the patient's condition is rapidly declining? Why, or why not?

As you begin to prepare for any test, review in your memory how your instructor talked about the information you have been learning. This will help you determine whether the test may focus more or less on memory and comprehension or on higher-level thinking such as application, analysis, and evaluation—or perhaps both. This will also help you know what kinds of test questions to expect.

For example, for memory and comprehension, usually objective test questions are used. These include multiple choice, true/false, and similar question types. Test questions focusing on higher-level understanding may also include objective questions but also likely include short-answer and essay questions. We'll look at all these types of questions in the next sections.

## Objective Tests

There is only one right answer for each question on an objective test. The point is to test your recall of facts. Most standardized tests are objective with one or more of these types of questions:

- multiple choice
- true or false

- short answer
- sentence completion
- problem solving

When taking an objective test, first look over the entire test to see how many questions there are. Try to answer them in order, but if you hit a difficult one, move on to the next. Just make sure you mark the tough question so you remember to come back to it. You can go back to the hard questions you marked when you've reached the end of the test and have extra time. Working on the easier questions first may help you answer the hard ones. Information from other questions might spark memories and prompt you to remember the answers.

## HOW TO DECIPHER MULTIPLE CHOICE QUESTIONS

There are certain guidelines to follow on a multiple choice test.

- Read each question carefully. Phrases like *except*, *not*, and *all of the following* provide important clues to the correct answer.

- Try to answer each question before you look at the answer choices. Then, try to match your answer to one of the choices. Even if you feel you have a match at choice one, read the rest of the choices to see if there's an even closer match.

- Use a process of elimination to narrow your answer choices. Some answers are clearly wrong. Cross them out and focus on the ones that might be correct.

- Work quickly! You won't have time to go back and answer truly hard questions if you take too long checking and double-checking the ones you think you answered correctly.

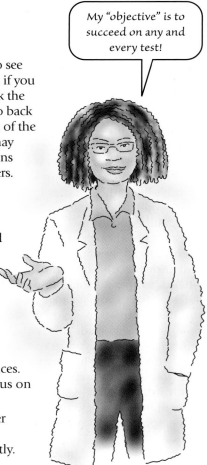

My "objective" is to succeed on any and every test!

---

### Who Decides What's *Best*?

You do! Sometimes, test instructions tell you to choose the "best" answer. That means more than one answer choice may technically be correct, but only one choice fully answers the question. You have to prioritize the answers to determine which best answers the question.

When you're prioritizing answer choices, use well-known theories or principles. For a question that asks what you would do first, for example, think of Maslow's hierarchy of needs. This theory basically says that although all needs seem important, they can be ranked. Needs at the bottom of the rankings can be dropped. In a well-written test, all answer choices seem plausible. No single choice stands out as obviously wrong. To apply Maslow's hierarchy to tests, you have to try and rank the choices. Look for a clue in the question that makes one answer better than the others. Sometimes, questions and answers are taken word for word from your textbook or lecture notes. If you recognize familiar words or phrases in only one of the options, that option is probably the right answer.

Be alert for "attractive distracters," or words that look like the correct answer but aren't. For instance, if *ileum* is the correct answer on an anatomy test, *ilium* might be included as another answer choice.

## TRUE OR FALSE?

In general, true/false questions are meant to see if you recognize when simple facts and details are misrepresented. Most true/false statements are straightforward and are based on key words or phrases from your textbook or lectures. Always decide whether the statement is completely true before you mark it as true. If it is only partly true, then the statement should be marked false. Statements containing extreme words can be tricky. Watch out for words such as the following:

- all
- always
- never
- none
- only

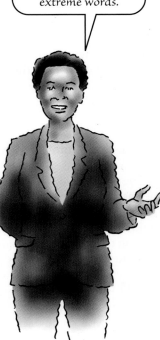

**Always** watch out for statements with extreme words.

## SHORT ANSWER

Short-answer questions are like the 100-meter dash of test items. These types of questions usually ask for one or two specific sentences, such as writing a definition or giving a formula. When you're taking a short-answer test, quickly scan the test items to organize them in three categories:

- answers I know without hesitation
- answers I can get if I think for a moment
- answers I really don't know

Answer the questions you know first and then move on to the questions that need a little thought. Once you're rolling and feeling confident, go for the tougher questions.

Note: most short-answer questions are objective questions, with only one correct answer. In some cases, however, a short-answer question may be subjective, allowing you to demonstrate your understanding through a variety of possible answers. Either way, just make sure your answer is clearly and concisely stated.

## FILLING IN THE BLANKS

Sentence completion or fill-in-the-blank questions usually ask you to supply an exact word or phrase from memory. Sometimes, you can use the length and number of blanks as a clue to the best answer. Many instructors will indicate whether they expect one word, two, or a phrase by using longer and shorter blanks. Also, make sure your answer is consistent with the grammar of the sentence. For example, if the question reads, "The medical term for heart muscle is _____ muscle," the answer should be *cardiac*, not *cardio* or *cardium*.

If you're really in doubt, go ahead and guess—you may receive partial credit.

Many times, the question itself will give clues to the right answer. For instance, a date may help you narrow the scope of answers by providing a historical point of reference. Suppose you think a scientific discovery might have been made by either Anton van Leeuwenhoek or Louis Pasteur and the date given is 1870. The right answer would have to be Pasteur because van Leeuwenhoek died in 1723.

## THE SOLUTION TO YOUR PROBLEMS

Problem-solving tests are most often found in subjects dealing with numbers and equations, such as math and science. With a problem-solving test, first read through all the problems before answering any of them. Underline key words in the directions and important data in the questions. Make notes next to any questions that bring thoughts or data points to mind. Then, go back and begin to fully answer the questions.

### What to Tackle First

Students often think they should start with the hardest problems so they can be sure those problems will be completed. They believe they can rush through the easy questions at the end. But it's actually better to start with the easy questions. They warm up your brain and build your confidence. Additionally, rushing to complete easy questions at the end can lead to careless mistakes and omissions.

### Moving On

If you have trouble solving a problem, move on. When you come back to that problem, take advantage of the fact that you've been working on

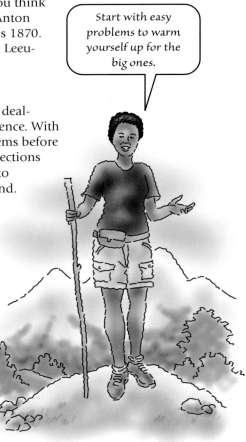

Start with easy problems to warm yourself up for the big ones.

something different and look at the old problem in a new way. Will any of the strategies or formulas you used on the other problems work? There's usually more than one way to solve a problem. If the strategy you started with isn't working, try something else.

> **Get It All Down**
>
> Show your work! If you make a mistake, the instructor will be able to see where you got off track and may give you partial credit. Also, when you write down all your work, you can check it yourself before you turn in the test. Checking your work helps you make sure you haven't made any careless errors or forgotten anything.

## Subjective Tests

In a subjective test, there's no single right answer. Instead, you're graded on how well you demonstrate your understanding of the material. Follow these steps for successfully completing essay tests.

- Read all the directions, underlining important words and phrases.
- Read all the questions, even if you're not required to answer them all. Jot down facts and thoughts for each question.
- Estimate how long you think you'll need to answer each question.
- Choose the questions you want to answer, when given a choice.
- Outline each answer.
- Write the answers.
- Review and proofread your answers. Then, reread the directions, making sure you followed them correctly.

Think about essays as endurance races. If completing a short-answer question is like running the 100-meter dash, then writing an essay is like running a 5-kilometer race. It just takes a little more thought and planning.

### LOOK BEFORE YOU LEAP

When you read all the directions in a test first, you reduce your chances of losing points by not following the directions. For example, the directions may ask you to provide three supporting facts for your statement. If you skip over that part of the directions, you might provide only one or two facts. When you're reading through the directions, underline the key points so you can refer to them with a glance as you write.

### Preview the Questions

Next, read through each question and make notes about any ideas or facts that come to mind. You can include things like formulas, names, dates, and your impressions. You'll need this information later as you create an outline. This step also helps you choose which questions to answer because it gives you an idea of how much you know about each topic.

### It's Just a Matter of Time

The next step is estimating how long it will take to answer each question. Consider things like the number of questions and how many points each question is worth. If one question is worth half the test grade, for example, plan to spend half your time answering it. Factor in things like the time you'll need to organize an outline, write the essay, and proofread your work.

## ORGANIZE AN OUTLINE

When you begin making an outline, start with your thesis statement. Choose a title that reflects your thesis and write it at the top of your paper. That way, you can use your title and thesis statement to guide your writing and keep it on track.

Content and organization typically count for most of the points on an essay test. The five-paragraph format is a good way to organize your information. (See *Five-Paragraph Format.*) If you run out of time and can't finish your essay, you can at least turn in your outline to let your instructor know that time was the problem, not comprehension.

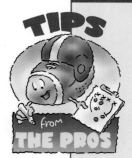

## Five-Paragraph Format

The five-paragraph format is an easy-to-follow structure for stating and supporting an opinion. It's a great way to get started on your essay, and it also helps you finish writing by taking the guesswork out of where to go next.

1. *Introduction.* Briefly outline your opinion and the facts you will use to support it.
2. *First point.* State your first point and include one to two supporting facts.
3. *Second point.* State your second point and include one to two supporting facts.
4. *Third point.* State your third point and include one to two supporting facts.
5. *Conclusion.* Pull together the three main points in a summary.

Note, however, that there's nothing magic about the number *three* for your key points! If you have only two main points to make, don't trump up some third thing just to have three in the body of your essay—that would just weaken your essay overall. Similarly, if you have a fourth key point to make, don't leave it out just because you think you *must* have five paragraphs. In other words, your essay should reflect what you actually have to say on the subject.

## FOLLOW YOUR GAME PLAN

When you're writing, stick to your outline to avoid wasting time. Your thesis statement should be a clear, but brief, answer to the essay question. In your introduction, explain what the remaining paragraphs in your essay will discuss. The essay question may ask you to "explain a cause-and-effect relationship" or "summarize key ideas." Be sure to follow directions here.

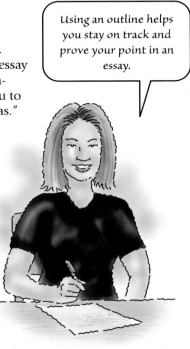

*Using an outline helps you stay on track and prove your point in an essay.*

Each paragraph in the body of the essay should make one point and support it with facts. This will help you be clear in your writing. There's no need to develop long, winding arguments. Go straight from point A to point B and give the facts that led you there. Avoid making several points in one paragraph or bringing in facts that don't really apply to your point or that you'll use later. Each paragraph should have a topic sentence that flows from your thesis statement. Write simple, direct sentences that follow one another logically.

In the conclusion, restate your thesis, then refer to the points you've made that prove it. Use the conclusion to draw your ideas together.

## Essay Tests Made Easy

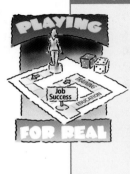

Hi, I'm Owen. I used to be very anxious about essay tests. I felt like I couldn't remember the main point I was trying to make—I got lost in the details. Now what I do is write my outline on a separate sheet of paper and I leave a lot of space between sections. Then I write one sentence that gives a fact to back up my point under each section in the outline. After that, I go back and write one more sentence with a fact under each section. I do this until I have four sentences under each section. Then I copy what I've written onto my test paper, adding any more details I can think of. This way, I know my essay won't be top-heavy at the start and rushed at the end and I stay on track with my main point.

## INSTANT REPLAY

When you're done writing, go back and read the question you've answered and the directions again. Make sure you've answered the question fully. Then review your essay for grammar errors and make sure your handwriting is legible. Make corrections where necessary.

---

### Essay Quick-Check

After completing an essay, check your work. Ask yourself these questions regarding the following three elements of your essay:

Content:

- Did I stick to my thesis statement?
- Did I prove each point I made?
- Did I use examples?
- Did I distinguish fact from opinion?
- Did I mention any exceptions to my general statements?

Organization:

- Did I open with my thesis statement?
- Does the thesis statement answer the question?
- Did I follow my outline?
- Does my conclusion pull together all my points?

Writing mechanics:

- Does every sentence make a clear point?
- Did I use all words correctly?
- Are spelling, grammar, punctuation, and sentence structure all correct?
- Is my work neat and my handwriting legible?

---

## Other Types of Tests

Other types of tests include:

- *Vocabulary.* These tests assess your ability to remember the meaning of a word and to use it correctly. They're used in foreign language courses or fields with specialized terminology.

- *Reading comprehension.* These tests require you to read a passage and answer questions about its content.

- *Open-book and take-home.* You're usually allowed to use any and all materials you want when taking these kinds of tests. Critical thinking is more important than a good memory here. However, there's less slack given for making factual errors.

- *Oral.* Speaking clearly and fluently is key here. If you can choose your topic in advance, do so and prepare like you were going to write an essay, with a thesis statement and outline. Try to make three points supported by facts.
- *Standardized.* The Graduate Record Examination (GRE) and Scholastic Assessment Test (SAT) are two examples of standardized tests. They are used for placement and admissions. Most tests required for certification or licensure in a health care career (discussed later in this chapter) are also standardized tests.

## VOCABULARY TESTS

Vocabulary tests call for some special strategies:

- Avoid decoy answer choices that look correct but aren't.
- Try to figure out if the word is a noun, verb, adjective, etc., and choose grammatically correct answers only.
- If you don't know the meaning of a word, try to remember where you've heard it and how it was used in the sentence. Select the answer that seems closest in meaning.
- Apply your knowledge of other languages. Prefixes, suffixes, and root words can offer clues about meaning.

## READING COMPREHENSION TESTS

These types of tests will go more smoothly if you read the questions first. Then, as you read the passage, you can focus on finding the information you need. Use only facts found in the passage! This is one case where applying outside knowledge is not helpful.

## OPEN-BOOK TESTS

Open-book tests also require special strategies:

- Use the index and table of contents to locate information.
- Avoid copying directly from your materials! Use as many resources as are allowed, but put ideas into your own words.
- Check your answers to make sure you didn't insert any incorrect information or unsupported arguments by mistake.
- As always, proofread your work!

## ORAL TESTS

Oral tests should be prepared for like written tests, with one twist: you should rehearse your answers out loud. Here are more strategies:

- Dress well and look neat. Stand up straight and look your listener(s) in the eye.
- Speak clearly and speak up. Don't go too fast or too slowly (rehearsal will help you with this).

- If you're giving a speech, prepare notes and rehearse speaking with only a few glances at your notes. Never read directly from your notes—your voice will be muffled and you won't make eye contact.

- Use your everyday language (except for slang) as much as possible. Using big or unfamiliar words will cause you to hesitate—and make mistakes.

- If you don't understand a question you get during or after your speech, ask for clarification. If you're still unsure, rephrase the question yourself.

- If you don't know the answer to a question, explain why. Perhaps it is outside your realm of expertise.

- When the test is over, gather your papers together and thank your audience for their attention.

Oral tests are much like presentations and public speaking. See the tips in Chapter 7.

## STANDARDIZED TESTS

Prepare for standardized tests by taking a practice test in similar testing conditions. Find a room that's free of distractions and allow yourself the same amount of time you'll have for the real test. The company that publishes the test likely provides practice questions or other study materials. If not, there are often published guides, like books and software, for each test. These guides contain practice exercises and self-tests.

These guidelines are true also for certification and licensure exams in many health care professions.

### Postgame Commentary

Reviewing your test after it has been graded can help you learn where you got off track and what you need to go over before the next test. When you get a corrected test back, ask yourself:

- Was there one concept or problem that tripped me up?

- How would I sum up the instructor's comments?

- Did I prepare adequately? How should I prepare differently next time?

- Did I make any careless mistakes? How can I avoid them next time?

- What can I learn from my mistakes?

## One Final Strategy

Tests give you an opportunity to evaluate how well you're doing in a course. Many instructors review tests with the entire class. One final test-taking strategy is to review your own test when it's given back to you. (See *Postgame Commentary.*) Try to learn from the comments your instructor made. If you have questions, make an appointment to see the instructor during office hours.

Remember, it's never good to argue with an instructor about your grade in class. But if you have questions or believe the instructor made an error in grading, approach the instructor privately—outside of class. Be sure to present your concerns in a respectful way.

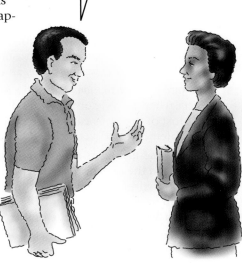

*Try talking with your instructor to get more information on how to improve your test performance.*

# SUCCEEDING ON MATH TESTS

Many students are especially anxious about math tests. But with good study habits and advance preparation, math tests should not be any more difficult than other types of tests.

Math questions generally fall into one of two categories: number questions and word problems. Both types involve solving problems and using math principles. Several strategies can be used to approach either type of test.

## Practice Tests

Take some practice tests to prepare for test day. Many textbooks include practice questions. You also can find many websites that offer practice tests—some created by instructors for their students using old tests! Take the test without looking at the answers and then grade yourself. You'll be glad you took practice tests when you sit down for your actual exam—they build your confidence and get you used to performing under test conditions.

## Number Problems

Here are a few simple steps that can help you increase your likelihood of success when taking a number-problem test:

- *Work carefully and deliberately.* You can really sabotage yourself by being careless or working too fast. Thorough work is required.

Write carefully, perform the calculations in reverse to check your answer, keep numbers in straight columns, and copy accurately.

- *Write out all steps.* Sometimes, students feel that showing all their work is childish. But it's a good practice at any age. If you write out your work, you can catch errors in it more easily.

- *Estimate first.* Try to estimate the answer to a problem before you start working. Then, solve the problem without referring to the estimate. When you finish your calculations, compare your answer with the estimate to see how close they are. If they're not close, you may have made a mistake in your calculations—a decimal point in the wrong place, an extra zero, etc.

- *Make sure your calculations use all the information given in the problem.* There's rarely unnecessary data given in a math problem. Most of the time, each piece of data is essential to solving the problem.

- *Read each question twice.* After you think you have the right answer, read the question again. Use a mental checklist. Did you show your work? Did you answer in the correct units? Did you answer all parts of the question? Does your answer make sense? If your answers are yes, you're on the right track.

- *Be persistent.* Everyone gets stuck sometimes. There are ways you can get yourself moving again. Round fractions up to whole numbers to put a problem into simpler form. Try to figure out what information you think you're missing. What doesn't make sense? Where do you lose track? If all else fails, move on to other questions and come back to the tougher ones later.

## Avoiding Careless Mistakes

**TIPS** from **THE PROS**

Careless mistakes result when students speed through problems. To avoid these mistakes and increase your accuracy, follow these tips:

- Write your numbers carefully so your sevens don't look like ones or fours and your eights don't look like sixes or zeroes.

- Whether you're doing simple or elaborate calculations, keep your digits in straight columns. You don't want numbers in the tens column being counted in the hundreds column.

- If you copy a problem onto another page, double-check to make sure you copied it accurately. You'd be surprised how often you can overlook a silly mistake—like writing a subtraction sign instead of a division sign—and not even realize it.

# Word Problems

Word problems have a bad reputation for being difficult. But word problems simply put numbers in a nonnumber context. There are some things you can do to make word problems more approachable:

- Look at the big picture.
- Plan well.
- Use strategies for dealing with difficult word problems.
- Learn from past mistakes with similar problems.

## THE BIG PICTURE

When you're facing a test that includes word problems, look over the whole test first. As you read each problem, jot down notes in the margin about how you might solve it.

Work on the easiest problems first. Those are the problems where the solutions you should use are easy to identify. Solving easy problems first warms up your brain and builds confidence.

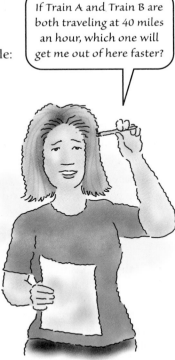

If Train A and Train B are both traveling at 40 miles an hour, which one will get me out of here faster?

## SET THE CLOCK

Consider planning for the test as you would plan time for a study session. Allow more time for problems worth more points. Budget time at the end of the test to review and to go back to difficult problems.

Those tough problems can derail your planning, but it doesn't have to be that way. Stay calm. Try not to give in to panic or feeling overwhelmed. There are several strategies you can use to solve tough problems:

- Mark key words and numbers, which can narrow the problem down to its essential elements.
- Sketch a diagram of the problem to make it more comprehensible.
- List all the formulas you think are relevant and decide which to use first.
- Think about similar practice problems and how you solved them.
- Guess at a reasonable answer if other strategies fail, then check it. If you can't work out the problem to get to your answer, you may think of another solution.

## LEARN FROM YOUR MISTAKES

After the test is over and you get it back from the instructor, read through the comments and suggestions. Try to avoid making assumptions about why you missed certain problems. Assumptions like "I just can't do math" or "It's just too hard" are unhelpful and counterproductive. Instead, ask yourself these questions:

- Did I make careless mistakes?
- Did I misread questions?
- Did I miss the same kind of problem over and over?
- Did I remember formulas incorrectly or incompletely?
- Did I run out of time?
- Did I practice enough or did I skimp on practice problems?
- Did I let my anxiety get the best of me, making me miss problems I really know how to solve?

Based on your answers to these questions, you can identify ways to improve your performance on future tests.

# CALCULATING GRADES

One of the reasons many students are anxious about tests is that they generally contribute heavily to the grade for the whole course. It's important, therefore, to understand how much any given quiz or test counts toward your grade and to be able to calculate your current grade status regardless of which of varying systems your instructor may use. Calculating your grade involves looking at what activities—tests, quizzes, homework, papers, etc.—earn points and how much each counts toward your final grade. Your syllabus usually provides this information.

In this section we'll describe how to calculate grades for point systems, averages, and weighted grade systems.

## Understanding Grades

Your instructor might assign a number of points or percentage values to each activity on the syllabus. If your instructor uses a point-based system, the easiest way to determine your grade is to convert the points to percentages. For example, if you take a test and receive a score of 40 out of 50 possible points (40/50), you can convert this score to a percentage to figure out your grade on the test. When figuring out percentages, remember to divide the number of points you received by the total number of possible points. A score of 40/50 equals 80%.

At any point during a semester or term, you also should be able to figure out your overall grade in a course. Let's say your syllabus lists the following information:

- Five quizzes—worth 40 points each
- Test 1—worth 100 points
- Test 2—worth 200 points

So far, the class has taken one quiz and Test 1, for a total of 140 possible points (40 + 100 = 140). After adding up the points you received on the quiz and test, you find that you have a total of 120 out of 140 possible points (120/140). Based on this information, you can figure out your overall percentage grade.

$$120 \div 140 = 85.7\%$$

If you keep track of your quiz and test scores (as well as any other graded activities) throughout the term, you'll be able to determine your overall grade in a course at any time. Knowing your grade in each course can help you gauge whether or not you're on target to meet your goals. Also, by keeping tabs on your grades, you can react early if they begin to slip. You may realize that you need to put in more study time, meet with your instructor, or visit the tutoring center. But if you wait until the end of the semester to figure out your overall grade in a course, it may be too late to improve it!

> To find your "batting average" in a course, just add up your scores and divide by the number of activities that have been assigned so far.

## Batting Averages

Now let's look at a grading system based on *averages*. Suppose your instructor says that the average of six test grades will be your final grade in the course. By the middle of the term, the class has taken three tests. For example, if your test grades were 78%, 91%, and 95%, what would your overall grade be so far? Follow these simple steps to determine your average grade.

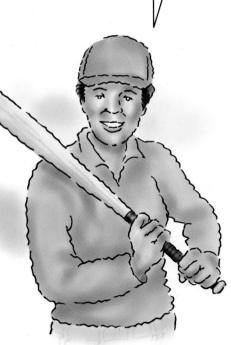

1. First, add your three test scores (78 + 91 + 95 = 264).
2. Then, divide the total by the number of tests you've taken so far (264 ÷ 3 = 88).

This means your grade in the course would be 88%.

## Weighting

In some cases, each activity listed on a syllabus is *weighted*, or assigned a certain percentage of the final grade. This means some activities will affect your final grade more than others, as shown below.

- Five quizzes—each is worth 10% of your final grade
- Test 1—worth 20% of your final grade
- Test 2—worth 30% of your final grade

Let's analyze these percentages. At first glance, it looks like the quizzes are not worth as much as Test 1 or Test 2. But look more closely; the syllabus says that *each* quiz is worth 10% of your final grade, which means:

$$5 \text{ quizzes} \times 10\% = 50\%$$

Therefore, the quizzes will make up 50% or half of your final grade. That's a big difference from 10%!

---

### When Projects, Papers, and Homework Are in Play

Many instructors also include activities such as projects, papers, homework, and participation in a student's final grade. Let's look at a scenario with several weighted activities.

- Four quizzes—each is worth 5% of your final grade
- Test 1—worth 10% of your final grade
- Test 2—worth 20% of your final grade
- Group project—worth 5% of your final grade
- Homework—worth 5% of your final grade
- Attendance and participation make up the rest of your grade

Now, which is most important? You might think the quizzes or tests are more important to your final grade than your attendance and participation. Look more closely.

- Quizzes are 20% of your final grade (4 quizzes × 5% = 20%).
- The tests together equal 30% of your grade (10% + 20% = 30%).
- The group project plus homework equal 10% of your grade (5% + 5% = 10%).

That leaves 40% for your attendance and participation—the largest percentage of all!

---

## Calculating Your Stats

So how do you figure out your grade in a course where the activities are weighted? Let's determine a student's grade based on the following syllabus information.

- Quizzes—average of six quizzes is worth 15% of your final grade
- Test 1—worth 25% of your final grade
- Test 2—worth 60% of your final grade

Suppose a student averaged all of her quizzes for a score of 70%. On Test 1, her grade was 80% and on Test 2, she received a score of 90%. How can we determine her final grade in the course if the activities are all weighted differently?

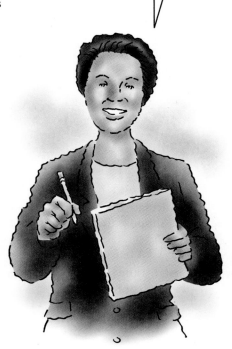

Keep track of your stats in each course by recording your scores when your instructor hands back graded assignments.

1. First, take all three scores and multiply each by the appropriate percentage, as listed on the syllabus. This will give each score the correct weight.

   Quizzes—70(.15) = 10.5

   Test 1—80(.25) = 20

   Test 2—90(.60) = 54

2. Next, add the three products you came up with in step 1.

   10.5 + 20 + 54 = 84.5

3. The sum is the student's overall grade in the course: 84.5%.

## Grading Scales

It's no use knowing how many points you earned or what your grade averages were if you're unable to translate that information into a letter grade. Here's a sample grading scale from a syllabus:

97−100 = A+

94−96 = A

90−93 = A−

86−89 = B+

83−85 = B

80−82 = B−

76−79 = C+

73−75 = C

70−72 = C−

66−69 = D+

63−65 = D

60−62 = D−

59 and under = F

For example, if a student received an overall grade of 84.5% in a course, that would translate to a B.

Many schools use the 4.0 system to calculate student grade point averages (GPAs). To do this, they assign point values to each student's letter grades. Here's a sample list based on the 4.0 system:

A+ = 4.3

A  = 4.0

A− = 3.7

B+ = 3.3

B  = 3.0

B− = 2.7

C+ = 2.3

C  = 2.0

C− = 1.7

D+ = 1.3

D  = 1.0

D− = 0.7

F  = 0.0

Let's calculate the GPA of a student who has completed one semester. Suppose this student took four three-credit courses during his first semester. His overall grades were A, B+, A+, and C−. What would his GPA be?

1. First, list the point values assigned to each of the letter grades the student received.

   A  = 4.0

   B+ = 3.3

   A+ = 4.3

   C− = 1.7

2. Next, find the average of the four point values.

   4.0 + 3.3 + 4.3 + 1.7 = 13.3

   13.3 ÷ 4 = 3.325

3. The average is the student's GPA: 3.325 (which, rounded to the nearest decimal point, comes to 3.3).

Keep in mind that the 4.0 system varies from school to school. For example, certain courses may be weighted more than others. You can talk to your academic advisor if you have questions about the system your school uses.

## The Home Stretch

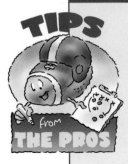

Suppose you're in the home stretch—the term is almost over and you just have one more biology test to take. You'd really like to reach your goal of getting a B in the course, but you're not sure if that's possible. What grade would you have to get on the last test in order to get a B in the course?

1. First, look at the syllabus to see how much each graded activity is worth. For example, suppose your syllabus lists this information:

   - Five quizzes—average of 5 quizzes is worth 20% of your final grade
   - Test 1—worth 30% of your final grade
   - Test 2—worth 50% of your final grade

2. Next, list your scores for each activity. Let $x$ stand for the score of your last test, since you haven't taken it yet. For the sake of this example, we'll use the following scores:

   Quizzes—70%

   Test 1—75%

   Test 2—$x$

3. Then, take all three scores and multiply each by the appropriate percentage, as listed on the syllabus. This will give each score the correct weight.

   Quizzes—$70(.20) = 14$

   Test 1—$75(.30) = 22.5$

   Test 2—$x(.50) = .5x$

   > A simple equation can help you figure out how to achieve your goal grade in a course.

4. Now, add the three products you came up with and make the sum equal to 80, as below. (This will be a basic algebraic equation used to find the value of $x$.) The value of $x$ is the percent grade you will need to get on the test in order to receive a B (or at least 80%) in the course.

   $14 + 22.5 + .5x = 80$

   $36.5 + .5x = 80$

   $36.5 + .5x - 36.5 = 80 - 36.5$

   $.5x = 43.5$

   $.5x \div .5 = 43.5 \div .5$

   $x = 87$

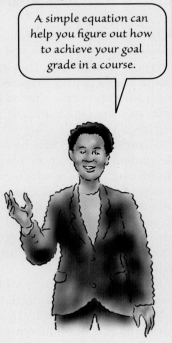

5. And you have your answer! In order to receive a B in the course, you'd have to score at least 87% on the last test.

## Grade Calculation Practice

At the midpoint in a semester, suppose a student has received the following scores:

- Quizzes—8/10, 6/10, 9/10, 10/10
- Homework assignments—5/5, 4/5, 3/5, 5/5
- Research paper—139/150
- Midterm exam—184/200

Based on the information above, calculate the following percentages (check your answers in the Appendix):

1. Assuming that each activity is weighted equally, what is the student's overall grade in the course so far?
2. What is the student's average quiz grade?
3. What is the student's average homework grade?
4. What percentage grade did the student receive on the research paper?
5. What percentage grade did the student receive on the midterm exam?

## CERTIFICATION AND LICENSURE EXAMS

> If you have the option, becoming certified in your field is one of the best ways to get your new career off to a great start.

After you complete your educational program, to enter many health care careers, you may be required to take a licensure examination. This is a test mandated by state law to ensure you are prepared to practice in your field. Such a licensure examination is used in most professions, the same as a law school graduate having to pass the bar exam before practicing law.

Certification may also be required or may be an option for you, depending on your chosen health career and your state. In most health care careers in which certification is available but is voluntary, it is still a good idea to become certified because this usually makes it easier to find the kind of job you want and to advance within your career. Certification, like licensure, requires an examination after completing your educational program. Certification is usually controlled by a professional association.

Because there are literally hundreds of specific health careers with their own legal requirements for licensure (which may vary by state) and different associations controlling certification, it is impossible to tell you *exactly* what to expect from these exams in your specific field. But you can easily find out yourself, and we can generalize about most licensure and certification exams. Follow these guidelines:

- Don't wait until you're almost finished with school before thinking about an upcoming licensure or certification exam. You should find out at the start of your program what the certification requirements are for your profession. Start by asking an instructor about what exam(s) you will need or want to take.

- Visit the website of your state's licensing agency and the professional association that administers the certification exam. Print out the basic information and highlight things like when the exam is given, when and how to register for the exam, what the exam covers, and the type of questions on the exam.

- Pay special attention to the test itself and the testing situation. Most such exams are multiple choice and some are given only on computers at the test site.

- Plan a study schedule well in advance of the exam, reviewing your educational materials related to topics you can expect on the exam. Use the study strategies described earlier in this chapter and in Chapter 8.

- Prepare for the type of test as described earlier in this chapter, such as how to perform best on multiple choice tests.

- Practice exams (and often review books with practice exams) are available in almost all health care fields where licensure or certification requires an exam. Taking one or more practice exams well before the test date will help you see if you need to study certain areas more and will give you confidence for the actual exam.

- Keep the exam in mind throughout your school program. Hang on to materials that you think will help you study for the exam when the time comes.

## CHAPTER SUMMARY

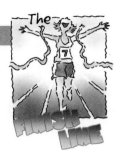

- Help reduce test stress by taking care of your body by exercising, eating right, and getting enough rest.

- Meet stress head-on with relaxation techniques, positive thinking, and by relying on your support network.

- Give yourself time to prepare and plan for tests. Talk with your instructor about what to expect, create a study plan, and take practice tests.

- With all kinds of tests, always read the directions and skim through the questions before you begin.

- When taking objective tests, work on the easier questions first to warm up your brain and jog your memory.
- For subjective tests, create an outline to help you get started on your essay.
- Review all graded tests to see where you can make improvements.
- Begin preparing well ahead for a licensure or certification exam, and take a practice test or two to ensure you've mastered the material and are confident for test day.

## REVIEW QUESTIONS

1. Short Essay: Write three to five sentences describing how to fight test anxiety.
2. How can you find out more about an upcoming test?
3. Short Essay: Write three to five sentences describing how to write an outline for an essay and why doing so is important.
4. List some tips for doing well on multiple choice questions, whether on a class test or licensure exam.

## CHAPTER ACTIVITIES

1. Exercise Checklist: Review *Health and Stress Management*. Choose the types of exercise and/or relaxation techniques you wish to do on a regular basis to minimize your stress and test anxiety and make a note of what you'll have to do to get started.
2. Test-Taking Exercise: Divide into groups of three. Each group member will come up with a five-question test for this course. The questions can be multiple choice, sentence completion, true/false, etc., or a mixture of question styles. Arrange a time to meet for 1 hour. Each of you will take a test you didn't write and complete it in 20 minutes. For the rest of the hour, go over the tests as a group, helping each other see where you made mistakes or did well. Discuss the strategies you used to answer the different types of test questions.
3. Looking Ahead Activity: Find out whether you will be taking a licensure exam after finishing your education and visit the website of the licensing agency to learn about the exam.

# ENTERING
# A HEALTH
# PROFESSION

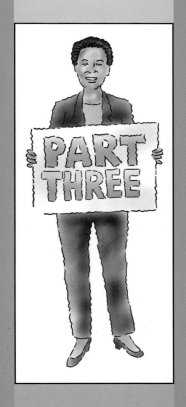

## CHAPTER 10

# Preparing for Your Career Path

## WINNING STRATEGY

*On completion of this chapter and the learning activities you will be able to:*

- Understand the basic groups of different health care careers

- Find detailed information about health careers in which you may be interested

- Identify your personality traits and interests as they relate to health careers

- Describe the personal characteristics needed for working successfully in a health profession

- Recognize the importance of professional conduct

- List the characteristics of a profession

You may already be registered in a health career educational program and have already determined what courses you'll be taking as you prepare for a health profession. You may have chosen your career—or at least an area of health care you're interested in working in. Even so, students sometimes change their career choices as they learn more about what's involved in education and training and what they would actually do on the job. Other students are still in the process of choosing. And all students should know what they'll be getting into in the future! This chapter will help you better understand different kinds of health care careers and the personal and professional traits needed.

# THE HEALTH PROFESSIONS

*Who* do you think of when you think about health care? Although many people answer doctors and nurses, at this point in your education you know about some of the many other health professionals also involved in health care. But did you know there are over 300 different health care careers? That's a lot to choose from!

Fortunately, you don't have to learn about all 300 different careers to find the career that best matches your interests and skills. Here's a good way to get started:

1. Learn about basic health care career groups.

2. Consider the education and training needed for possible careers.

3. Consider your personality and what you think you would like to do in your career. What personality traits and skills do you need to succeed in a health given care career? Take a self-assessment inventory to see how well you will fit in different professions.

4. Talk with academic advisor about your choices.

5. Confirm your choice and commit to your educational path.

> Be sure your chosen health career is a perfect fit for you.

## Health Career Groupings

Let's start with the basic groups of health careers. The National Consortium for Health Science Education (NCHSE), an organization of educators, has organized the 300 different health professions into five main groups. This is a good starting point for thinking about what different health professionals do in their work. (See *Examples of Health Care Careers* for additional examples of careers in these groupings.)

- *Therapeutic Services.* Health professionals who work in therapeutic services deliver health care directly to patients. In addition to physicians, nurses, and dentists, these careers include physician assistants, respiratory therapists, surgical technicians, dental assistants, home health aides, medical assistants, massage therapists, pharmacy technicians, and many others. People who work in these careers usually enjoy working directly with patients and helping them regain or maintain their health.

- *Diagnostics Services.* Professionals working in diagnostic services work closely with those in therapeutic services and often also are in direct contact with patients. Diagnostic health services, however, involve determining the nature of the patient's health problem, often using the latest technology. Examples of careers in diagnostic services are lab technicians, radiologic technologists, ophthalmic assistants, electrocardiographic (ECG) technicians, computed tomography (CT) technologists, and many others. People who work in these careers usually enjoy working with scientific equipment and technology and knowing their work will help identify patients' health problems so that they can receive the appropriate therapy.

- *Health Informatics.* Health informatics careers generally involve managing patient and other information—a crucial aspect of health care. Examples of these careers are health information management technicians, medical coders, medical transcriptionists, patient account technicians, and many others. Because most medical information is now managed with computerized systems, people who work in these careers usually enjoy working on a computer, using written language, and close attention to detail, often working independently. Although these careers typically involve less direct patient contact, they are a very important part of the health care team.

- *Support Services.* Many other health professionals contribute to the working of health care institutions and the full provision of health care. The general category of support services includes careers such as dietetic technicians, social workers, facilities managers, food safety specialists, and many others. These careers may or may not involve direct patient contact and vary widely in terms of responsibilities and educational training.

- *Biotechnology Research and Development.* Because science and technology are continually developing new approaches within health care, many careers involve research. A few examples are lab technicians, research assistants, and quality control technicians. Individuals in these careers, which often involve little patient contact, enjoy being part of a team focusing on science and the latest technology while they investigate new aspects of health care.

## Examples of Health Care Careers

### *Therapeutic Services*

- Anesthesiologist Assistant
- Athletic Trainer
- Audiologist
- Certified Nursing Assistant
- Dental Assistant
- Dental Hygienist
- Dental Lab Technician
- Dentist

### Examples, cont.

- Dietician
- Dosimetrist
- Emergency Medical Technician (EMT)
- Home Health Aide
- Licensed Practical Nurse
- Massage Therapist
- Medical Assistant
- Occupational Therapist
- Occupational Therapy Assistant
- Pharmacy Technician

- Physical Therapist
- Physical Therapy Assistant
- Physician
- Physician Assistant
- Recreation Therapist
- Registered Nurse
- Respiratory Therapist
- Speech Language Pathologist
- Surgical Technician
- Veterinarian Technician

### Diagnostic Services

- Cardiovascular Technologist
- Clinical Lab Technician
- Computed Tomography (CT) Technologist
- Cytotechnologists
- Diagnostic Medical Sonographers
- Electrocardiographic (ECG) Technician
- Electronic Diagnostic (EEG) Technologist
- Exercise Physiologist

- Histotechnician
- Magnetic Resonance Imaging (MRI) Technologist
- Medical Technologist
- Nuclear Medicine Technologist
- Pathology Assistant
- Phlebotomist
- Positron Emission Tomography (PET) Technologist
- Radiologic Technologist/ Radiographer
- Sonographer

### Health Informatics

- Admitting Clerk
- Community Services Specialists
- Data Analyst
- Health Educator
- Health Information Coder
- Health Information Services
- Medical Biller

- Patient Financial Services
- Medical Information Technologist
- Medical Librarian
- Reimbursement Specialist (HFMA)
- Transcriptionist
- Utilization Manager

## Examples, cont.

### Support Services

- Biomedical/Clinical Technician
- Central Services
- Environmental Health and Safety
- Environmental Services
- Facilities Manager
- Food Service
- Hospital Maintenance
- Industrial Hygienist
- Materials Management
- Transport Technician

### Biotechnology Research and Development

- Bioinformatics Associate
- Biostatistician
- Clinical Data Management Associate
- Clinical Trials Research Associate
- Lab Assistant
- Lab Technician
- Manufacturing Technician
- Product Safety Associate
- Processing Technician
- Quality Control Technician
- Research Assistant

# Learn More About Career Possibilities

With a general idea about one or more careers you may be interested in, it's easy to learn more about those specific professions. Your school likely has a student career office with directories and other books with detailed information about health care careers. Look for this information:

- Career titles
- Description of activities and roles performed
- Settings in which these professionals may work
- Education and training required
- Future job prospects and salary range

## GO ONLINE!

Information about specific health careers is also available online. The American Medical Association (AMA) website includes a Health Care Careers Directory that provides detailed information about more than 80 of the most popular health careers. Start at http://www.ama-assn.org/ama/pub/education-careers/careers-health-care/directory.shtml.

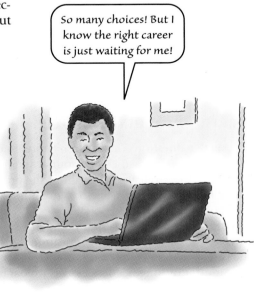

So many choices! But I know the right career is just waiting for me!

The U.S. Department of Labor, Employment and Training Administration maintains the "CareerOneStop" website with a wealth of information about many health careers. Start here: http://www.careeronestop.org/StudentsandCareerAdvisors/ ExploreCareersStudents.aspx and click on "Occupation Profile" to reach a list of careers with detailed information. This site can also tell you about the career facts in your own state. You can even see videos of people in many health careers doing their work.

# EXPLORING MAJORS FOR HEALTH CARE CAREERS

Assuming you are already enrolled in an educational institution, the best way to learn more about preparing for a health career is to start with your school's catalog. You may have a printed catalog, or it may be posted on the school's website. In addition, individual departments and programs often post descriptions of the coursework for majors and certificate programs for working in different careers. Pay attention to information such as:

- Prerequisites—courses or special background needed to enter the major or program
- The number of courses or terms to fulfill degree or program requirements
- Clinical experience required (usually through clinical labs or courses)
- Options such as elective courses in other areas of your interest
- The total number of terms and the associated costs of your education/training
- Additional education needed later on to advance your career options

## Making Academic Choices

If you have questions or still aren't sure exactly what career path interests you the most, talk to your academic advisor or department representatives to learn more about the program or major. This is one of the most important decisions you'll make in your life, so don't decide too quickly!

One of the first things many students notice about health care careers is the wide variety in educational preparation. Depending on the career, and your state's requirements for education and training, the amount of time needed for this preparation can vary from 1 year to 4 years of school, or more. When making your choice, however, the consideration of time should not be the key deciding factor. Instead, think about what you'll actually be doing in your future career and how much you will enjoy it. Your choice may determine how you'll spend many years or even all of your life! Although you can always change careers at some later time, that might mean returning to school at additional cost.

It's also important to think about how your career might evolve over time. Will you be happy doing the same work for as long as 20 or 30 years? Does your chosen career allow you to move up a ladder within the same profession, taking on new responsibilities and challenges? This is called a "career path" because your education and your first job after school are only the first steps on a path that may take you onward and upward in your chosen profession. As you work within your profession, you continue to gain new skills and learn new knowledge, allowing you to take on new responsibilities. You might become a supervisor and manage others who do what you once did. With experience or additional education, you may move up the ladder from an assisting role to take on a higher position or one with more independent functions.

If you're not sure where you can go in the future within a profession, talk to your advisor about this dimension of your choices as well.

## One Size Doesn't Fit All!

People who are happiest in their work usually feel their career matches their personality and interests perfectly. They enjoy going to work because it's something they like to do and consider it a profession, not just a way to earn a living, or a job.

But how can you know what career is perfect for you? The process begins with understanding yourself.

### KNOW YOURSELF

You already know a lot about yourself, even if you may not yet know everything about the health career in which you're interested. To get started, think about questions like these:

- Do you like working with people?
- Do you like helping people?
- Are you emotionally upset by the sight of blood, body fluids, or illness?
- Do you prefer being a team player or working independently?
- Are you more interested in the "human" side or the scientific side of health care?

- Can you work at a computer or lab bench for a long period without becoming restless?
- Do you enjoy communicating with others—whether by talking or writing?
- Do you like working with your hands?
- Do you prefer daily routines or frequently changing activities?
- Do you like solving problems?
- Do you like learning new things frequently?

These are just a few of the ways people differ. There are no right or wrong answers to any of these questions. But certain personality traits fit in better with some careers more than others. Your goal is to find the perfect fit for you.

If you're still not sure, even after you have learned about specific careers and their educational requirements, an inventory of your personality and interests may be just what you need to help you decide. Remember the different learning styles from Chapter 5? There you thought about how you best learn new information and skills. Do you learn more by seeing, hearing, or doing? Which kinds of learning activities are you most comfortable with? This can help you better understand your "career style" as well.

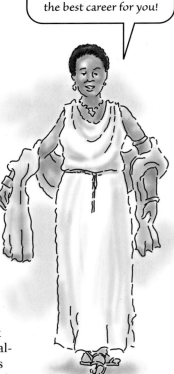

The ancient Greeks have always said, "Know thyself." That's how to find the best career for you!

## PERSONALITY AND INTERESTS INVENTORIES

Many schools have assessment tools to help students discover what specific career choices may be best for them, based on their personality and interests. These assessments usually ask a series of questions and then analyze your answers and suggest likely career matches. Ask your advisor if such a tool is available for you.

Self-assessment tools like these are also available online. Be careful when browsing the Internet, however, because many assessment sites will try to get you to pay for an assessment or other services! One good resource is the Careerlink Inventory, available free at http://www.mpcfaculty.net/CL/climain.htm. You will be asked to rate yourself and your interests (including preferred working conditions and career preparation time) and then you will receive an analysis you can print out of careers that may be a perfect match for you along with links directly to Web pages with information about those specific careers.

Here's how it works:

1. Start at http://www.mpcfaculty.net/CL/climain.htm

2. Answer the questions in the specific categories: Aptitudes, Interests, Temperaments, Physical Capacities and Working Conditions, and Career Preparation Time.

3. You then receive your Career Inventory Results listing, with a numerical match for different career clusters. Look for career clusters in the "Health Sciences" career area, and click on a health science "cluster title" in the column on the right.

4. This brings you to a screen of general information about careers in that grouping and a list of "sample occupations." Here you will find many health care careers that closely match your personality and interests.

5. Click on any of these occupations to be taken to the U.S. Department of Labor Web page for that career, where you can learn much more about the nature of the work, the education and training required, the outlook for the future in that profession, typical earnings, and other information.

Allow 10 minutes to take this survey online, plus some time to explore the career information to which you will be led. Not only may you learn something new about yourself, but you'll have some fun with this experience too!

## PERSONAL AND PROFESSIONAL TRAITS AND SKILLS

As you prepare to enter a health care profession, it's good to be thinking about what it means to be a professional. Having a career in a health profession is much more than simply working a job. To be a professional involves demonstrating certain characteristics and behaving in certain ways. This begins with who you are as a person, your personality traits.

## Personal Characteristics

When you work in health care, your personality and conduct really matter. Patients will probably see you face to face, whether you're providing direct care or taking their insurance information. They'll size up your character and make decisions about whether they can trust you and whether you seem to care about them. Your coworkers and other members of the health care team will do the same.

Patients also give you information that is very private—sometimes information not even their families know about. So you have to be the kind of person a patient can trust. Following are the main characteristics you need to have to be a good health care professional:

- *Caring.* Be someone who cares about the patients receiving health care.

- *Integrity.* Be recognized as someone who is honest and accountable and behave ethically.
- *Dependability.* Be someone who always accepts your responsibilities and works hard to meet the expectations for a professional in your position.
- *Trustworthiness.* Be someone who consistently does the right thing and is always honest.
- *Teamwork.* Be a willing and effective member of the health care team.
- *Openness to change.* Be flexible and willing to keep learning.
- *Personal health.* Be a model of good health habits and behaviors.

## CARING

It may seem obvious, but health care is all about caring for people's needs. Even if you're not in direct patient care—if you're working in a career behind the scenes—patients are still affected by the quality of your work. People who care about their work, who genuinely want to do their best, not only contribute more to the overall quality of health care but also are more successful in their career and experience more job satisfaction.

But caring begins now, as a student. Think about a student who only wants to get a passing grade on a test. This student may cram the night before the test and not be concerned if he or she forgets the material right after the exam. Now think about a student who really cares about his or her studies, understanding that in the future, actions taken on the job may be affected by how well one understands that material that was on the exam. A student who cares about learning, who sees the importance of learning for one's career, really wants to understand and be able to apply this knowledge or skill in the future.

Caring extends into all aspects of being a student. You should care enough to do your homework and assignments well and on time, to pay attention in class, to show respect for your instructors and other students.

Caring also means caring for other people—making the effort to understand their feelings. This kind of caring, known as empathy, is essential for health care professionals who work with patients. Empathy involves a felt concern for others that leads to a desire to help them. A caring person also is tactful, meaning that you consider the feelings of others before speaking in a way that might hurt another person.

## INTEGRITY

Integrity refers to the quality of your character. The character you develop as a student will influence the character you'll have as a health care professional. That's why it's important to start thinking about your character now, while you're in school.

People with integrity stand by their personal and professional codes of ethics. They're honest in everything they do and accept accountability for their actions. This quality is especially important to have as a health care professional. Someone with integrity will be sure to keep patient information private and will be honest about his or her actions—even after making a mistake.

## DEPENDABILITY

Dependability is crucial in health care. Medical facilities are busy places, which makes teamwork necessary for everyday office operations. Even one person not showing up to work or coming late can throw off the entire day. As a member of the health care team, you need to be there—your teammates are counting on you! Be someone who always makes it in to work on time.

Dependability also applies to the quality of your work. If you're asked to perform a task, you should always perform it when you are told to and to the exact specifications you are given. In the often hectic world of the health care facility, delays and mistakes add up to late hours and unhappy patients, or potentially worse outcomes.

Being dependable means that you'll always follow through and do what you're asked. It means that your coworkers, supervisors, and patients can feel comfortable putting their trust in you and relying on you to get the job done.

## TRUSTWORTHINESS

Being trustworthy means people can feel confident knowing you can be trusted in all situations and that you'll always do the right thing. Even as a health care professional, you may be tempted to cut corners or do things that are not quite on the up and up. Being trustworthy means you stand firm in your commitment to honesty, forthrightness, and doing things the right way. Not only will you feel good about yourself when you're trustworthy, but you'll also earn and keep the respect of everyone around you.

## TEAMWORK

Even while still a student, you're part of a team that includes instructors and other students. You will likely work on group projects with others, just as in your health career you will be part of a team providing or supporting patient care. To be an effective team player, you need to respect the other members of the team and what they have to offer. You need to make the effort to understand their point of view rather than thinking you yourself are always right. Commit yourself to working with others and doing your fair share and avoid complaining if sometimes it seems you might be doing more than just your share.

Working with others also requires the quality of patience. Be tolerant and understanding of others who may not be as quick to act. Being accepting helps you avoid feeling frustrated if things aren't going exactly as you'd prefer.

## OPENNESS TO CHANGE

Health care is continually evolving as new technology and new diagnostic and therapeutic approaches develop and the health care system itself changes. To succeed in this world of change, a professional must be flexible and always open to new learning. A rigid, unbending personality doesn't fit in well or adapt well when things change. Make an effort to stay open-minded and always willing to learn more. In fact, in health care more than in other professions, people take continuing education classes throughout their whole career so that they stay current in their field. This is very important so that you can remain current with new and emerging technology and procedures.

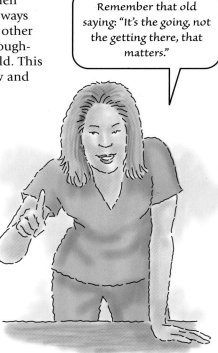

Remember that old saying: "It's the going, not the getting there, that matters."

As a student now, you are learning many new things. Most important is your attitude, so that you always stay open to continuing to learn. Don't view your education as something you "have to get through" and then you're done with it. Accept that you'll always be learning, that this is simply part of being a health care professional, and learn to enjoy it! Once you relax and realize that education is an exciting benefit of having a health care career, not a "price to pay" or just a stage to go through to enter that career, you'll find you enjoy your daily life as a student more.

Openness to change also means being able to accept criticism from others. Your instructors, like supervisors in your career, will offer you feedback that is both positive and designed to help you improve in areas that need improvement. Try not to feel resentful but, instead, accept criticism gracefully and continue to learn.

## PERSONAL HEALTH

As a health care professional, you will work to help others stay or become healthy, and health promotion is a key aspect of everything you'll do. You will in fact be a model for others—family and friends as well as patients—and you should do your best to demonstrate good health habits yourself. That includes eating well and maintaining a healthy weight, exercising regularly, getting enough rest, and not using tobacco, drugs, or excessive alcohol. Not only is this important for your own health and well-being, but others will judge you in your career by your personal habits. Remember, people pay far more attention to what you *do* than what you say!

## Professional Conduct

As you develop the personal characteristics just described, you're learning also how to act as a professional. Being a successful health care provider isn't just about remembering the facts you learned in school. Doing your job well is not simply performing tasks exactly how you learned to do them. It's also about how you present yourself—with your conduct. The most knowledgeable person in the world will have trouble inspiring patients or coworkers with confidence if he or she seems rude, sarcastic, sloppy, or haphazard. Instead, we learn to behave like a professional.

Remember that as a health care professional, every aspect of your conduct is scrutinized. Patients have to feel that they can trust you to take care of them. Your coworkers need to be reassured that you're capable of carrying out your responsibilities. You have to present yourself as a responsible person who is focused on work.

For example, think back to doctors, nurses, and other health care providers you've come in contact with. How would you feel if they stood in the hall gossiping while you waited in the exam room? How would you feel if they seemed like they were rushing, irritated, or impatient? Health care demands a high standard of professional conduct from its members. Here are some additional general guidelines for professional conduct:

- *Act responsibly.* Follow the standards of practice in your work and take responsibility for your own actions. Admit failures and don't try to blame others if something goes wrong. Follow ethical standards in everything you do.

- *Accept diversity and practice tolerance for others.* A professional knows people have different ideas, feelings, customs, and behaviors and does not judge them because of differences. Give the best possible care to all patients.

- *Communicate carefully and effectively.* Use the skills described in Chapter 7 when talking to patients, coworkers, and other health professionals. Avoid slang, sarcasm, and gossip—and never, ever violate the confidentiality of patients. You'll learn more about confidentiality in the next chapter.

- *Show initiative.* If you see a problem, don't ignore it just because it may be outside your immediate work. Share your ideas if you see ways that things can be improved. Remember that in the health care team, everyone has an important role—and everyone can raise questions or offer ideas for the good of all.

## Characteristics of a Profession

How is a health care career more than just a job? What makes a career a profession, rather than just going to work every day?

You've probably already worked in an ordinary job in your life. You may have gotten the job without having a specialized education or advanced training. You may have done a day's work without having to think much about what you're doing. You may have just done what you were told to do and gone back to your "real life" after work. In many jobs you might not feel a lifelong commitment to the work or a real enthusiasm that you were making a difference by applying all your knowledge, skills, and education in the performance of your duties. Although there's certainly nothing wrong with working such a job, you might not have felt completely satisfied by your work. Maybe that's why you've chosen to enter a health care career instead?

A profession, on the other hand, is more fulfilling because you are more completely involved—your work becomes part of who you are. Health care professions, like other professions, have a number of characteristics that make them different from ordinary jobs. As you move into your chosen career, you will participate increasingly in the profession, so it's a good idea to be thinking ahead about these characteristics. This will also help prepare you for your clinical experiences in your education, the subject of the next chapter. Even as a student you will likely very soon be in *real* health care practice!

### EDUCATION AND COMPETENCE

No one enters any profession without education and training to gain specialized knowledge and skills. As a student, you already know about the education required. Along with this comes the expectation that in your health care career you will have competence. That is, you have the knowledge and skills to do your work correctly and safely. It will not be necessary for a supervisor to stand over you at all times watching to make sure you're doing the right thing—you'll do your work well because you have learned how to do so and you care about it. That's one reason why it's important to care about your education now as a student. In the future you'll have the responsibility to act competently on your own when needed. It's a great feeling to know you can meet this challenge!

## SELF-REGULATING

Professions are generally said to be self-regulating. That means that even though the profession is in part governed by laws, the profession itself sets many of the standards by which people practice in it. For example, medical practice standards—such as the right way to perform medical procedures—are established by medical professionals. This makes good sense if you think about it: who other than the professionals in a field would know best about how their work should be done?

Professions are also self-regulating in terms of proper behavior. Most professions have an ethical code that spells out how people in that profession should act toward each other, their clients, and the general public. Health care professions also have ethical codes for how people in those careers should behave toward patients, coworkers, and others. In the next chapter you'll learn about the ethical codes of health professions.

## PROFESSIONAL ASSOCIATIONS

As one entering a health care career, you may already know about the one or more professional associations for practitioners in that career. A professional association is a nonprofit organization of people who work in a particular career, with many benefits for those who join. Most health care careers have professional associations and many allow students to become members so that they can begin receiving the benefits right away. A few of these benefits are:

- Subscriptions to professional publications
- Access to online resources
- Professional conferences, conventions, and workshops
- Information on new technologies
- Ethics guidelines
- Patient educational materials
- Networking opportunities
- Grant and scholarship opportunities

Once you have decided which career you are preparing for, take a few minutes to learn about its professional association. Ask your instructors or do an online search (search for "association + *name of career*"). Every association has a website and there you'll quickly learn what benefits you can begin receiving immediately that will help you even as a student become more professional as you move into your career.

## NETWORKING

Another important aspect of most professions is networking among the people in the profession. Networking is a process of developing relationships with other people with whom you share common interests and who may be helpful to you in your career. Most networking is done in an informal way. You might have a conversation with an instructor outside class and form a casual friendship after that course has ended. You might have expressed an interest in a particular type of work and maybe this instructor remembers this and later on tells you about a job opening he or she has learned about. That's networking in action. Or you might become friends with an older student who enters the profession ahead of you. If you stay in touch, you might one day learn of a particular internship from that person where he or she works. That's also networking. In reality, more jobs are filled by people who learned of an open position from someone they know than by people who respond to posted job openings.

Networking is not an attempt to use people, however. You shouldn't start networking motivated only by the thought of what you might get from them in the future. Rather, networking is more a matter of building friendships with people in your chosen field, whom you like and want to stay in touch with. You can start networking with other students right away. Forming a study group is a good way to spend time with other students in your career path. You get to know them as people at the same time you increase your knowledge and skills in your courses. Many lifelong friendships—and networks—begin during one's education years.

Once you are practicing in your profession, your network continues to be valuable. You talk to people in your network about your work and learn new things about the field. You can problem-solve together. And you always have people to whom you can turn if you need advice for any work-related issues that may occur.

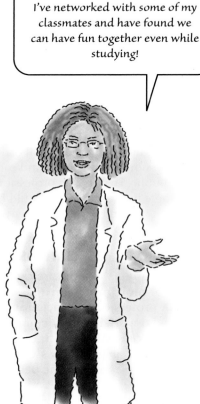

*I've networked with some of my classmates and have found we can have fun together even while studying!*

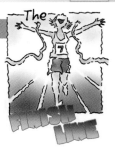

## CHAPTER SUMMARY

- Consider the five main groups of health care careers to determine or confirm which are most suitable for you.

- Research your chosen career through the Internet and resources available at your educational institution. Talk with your advisor if you have any questions.

- Use a self-assessment tool to explore your personality traits and personal interests to be sure your chosen career is a good match.

- Understand the personal characteristics that are important for working in a health profession. During your time as a student, work on developing your own characteristics and abilities so that you enter your career prepared to do your best.

- Accept what it means to be a professional. Conduct yourself in a way that inspires the trust and confidence of coworkers and patients.

- Begin participating in your profession right away through a professional association.

- Networking with others in your profession helps you get started and offers many benefits.

## REVIEW QUESTIONS

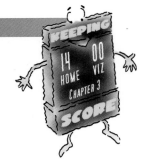

1. Which main group of health care careers interests you the most?

2. What is the employment outlook for your chosen career?

3. Describe your personality traits and interests that match up with your chosen career.

4. List at least five personal characteristics that are important in all health professions.

5. Name three characteristics of a profession.

## CHAPTER ACTIVITIES

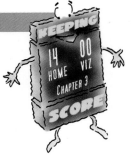

1. Online Exercise: Go to the U.S. Department of Labor website and look up a career in which you are interested in the Occupational Outlook Handbook. To search by an alphabetical index of all careers, start here: http://www.bls.gov/oco/ooh_index.htm. Or you can type in a career title to search for it here: http://www.bls.gov/search/ooh.htm. Read the section "Nature of the Work" to make sure people in this career do what you initially thought they do. Then read other information about that career you're interested in.

2. Group Discussion: With two or three other students, spend a few minutes talking about what you think are the most important personal characteristics for working in health care. Be sure each

person has the opportunity to speak. Then compare your responses and talk about *why* each characteristic is important. As a group, try to come up with an example of a patient care problem that could occur if someone on the health care team did *not* manifest that characteristic in their work.

3. Role Playing and Discussion: In groups of two to four students, devise a role play for a patient care interaction. The health care provider(s) in this role play should demonstrate either professional or unprofessional behavior in the interaction with the patient. After each role play, other students should critique the behavior observed and provide rationales for how they evaluate this behavior.

## CHAPTER 11

# Clinical Rotations

*On completion of this chapter and the learning activities you will be able to:*

- Embrace new skills in a clinical environment

- Ward off anxiety and stress

- Meet the standards of professionalism

- Preserve patient confidentiality and protect patient rights and safety

- Work in a culturally diverse environment

- Create a high standard of personal conduct

- Plan ahead for your clinical rotation

In this chapter, you'll look ahead to your clinical rotation or externship, which in many health care educational programs is the first step toward a new career. This is an exciting time! You'll learn about the professional standards of conduct you'll be expected to meet and about the importance of protecting patient rights and privacy. You'll also prepare for handling changes in your schedule and you'll learn how your clinical instructor can help you before and after you begin your rotation. This chapter will provide you with important information that will help you make your clinical rotation a positive experience.

First, a note about terminology. The phrase "clinical rotation" is typically used when the clinical learning experience is part of the school's integral academic program. The term "externship" is often used for a similar clinical learning experience that takes place outside the school's program. One or the other is usually required as part of the academic training for health care careers that have a clinical component. Although this chapter will use the phrase "clinical rotation," the basic principles apply equally in both situations.

# WELCOME TO THE REAL WORLD OF HEALTH CARE!

It's finally here: You're about to start your clinical rotation. You've probably imagined yourself in a health care setting, putting your knowledge into action. You've looked forward to this day—and maybe dreaded it a little, too. It's one thing to read about the tasks you'll be asked to perform, but quite another to actually carry out those tasks in the workplace. But this is an exciting opportunity to use your skills and begin to experience what your future career will really be like. Get ready to take full advantage of this experience!

*Jump right in! Experience will help you become more comfortable with the skills you'll use during your clinical rotation.*

## Embrace New Skills

You might feel that in your clinical rotation you'll be taking on many new responsibilities. But the only thing that's really "new" about the tasks you'll perform is the fact that you'll be doing them for the first time in a clinical setting. After all, you've read about these tasks, practiced them in the classroom or laboratory, and you already know what to do.

Of course, knowing what to do in your head is different than actually working with a patient or staff member. That's why it's a good idea to practice your skills on fellow students or even family members, whenever possible. Any skills involving needles and syringes or technical equipment need to be practiced in a supervised skills laboratory, of course.

### WELCOME TO THE LABORATORY

Many programs have students demonstrate certain skills in the laboratory before they perform these tasks during their clinical rotation. If you know there are certain tasks you'll be performing during your clinical experience and you'd like more practice, use the skills laboratory to brush up on them. Most schools have times when an instructor or student mentor works in the skills lab and provides assistance. Take advantage of those times to get extra help. If you're unsure how to get more practice, talk to your instructor.

### TAKE THE PLUNGE

Participating in skills labs will give you a good foundation for demonstrating skills during your clinical experience. Even so, it's natural to feel nervous the first time you actually have to do something in a real health care setting. You may feel like the only person in the room who hasn't performed a certain task a hundred times already. You might also feel like coworkers or patients are judging you unfairly for your inexperience.

The best way to get started with hands-on experience is to jump in. You may feel awkward at first or reluctant to ask a question (especially in front of a patient or coworker), but with repetition you'll gain valuable practical experience very quickly.

## Anxieties and Concerns

It's normal to be a little nervous about beginning a clinical experience. But even though it seems like an unknown, remember that you *are* prepared. This is what you've been working toward every day. And you won't be alone. Your clinical instructor or clinical mentor will be there to help you.

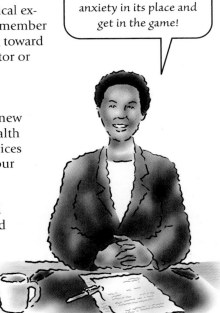

*Your clinical rotation is here—it's time to put anxiety in its place and get in the game!*

### YOU'RE NOT ALONE!

Although you're in a new environment, experiencing new things, you're not alone! Remember that all of the health care professionals you'll be working with were all novices at one time, too. You'll find camaraderie in sharing your experiences.

Your school may provide a clinical instructor to be with you during your clinical experience. Keep in mind that different programs may use different terms. Instead of a "clinical coordinator," you may have an "extern coordinator." Schools that do not send an instructor or coordinator to be with you usually arrange for someone on the job site to be your mentor. In either case, this person is there to help you and answer your questions.

### PUT ANXIETY IN ITS PLACE

Whether you'll be assisting with patients in the examination room, working in a lab, or handling medical coding and billing, you may feel some anxiety about doing the job. That's normal. If you ask people who are already working in health care, you'll probably find they felt the same way when they started out.

It's important to address and deal with your anxiety. Mild anxiety probably won't affect your performance on the job, but a high level of anxiety would be a distraction. The following tips will help you minimize anxiety if necessary:

- Use the relaxation techniques described in Chapter 3 to help relieve your anxiety.
- Make an appointment to see your clinical mentor or instructor. He or she can reassure you that what you're feeling is normal

and help you identify your anxieties and come up with a plan to reduce them.

- Take advantage of the resources offered by your school. Many schools also have counseling services that can help you cope with your stress.

## SCHEDULE OUT STRESS

As you think about starting your clinical rotation, you may also be concerned about its additional demand on your time. You've already pushed your schedule to the limits with school and work. Your clinical experience will require even more schedule changes. But you can manage these changes by knowing what to expect and how to prepare for them.

For example, remember the support network you have read about in earlier chapters. Family members, friends, classmates, and coworkers can all be sources of encouragement and support during your clinical experience. If you accept help from others during this busy time, you'll feel less stressed. (See *Your Safety Net: Family and Friends*.)

> During your clinical experience, you'll need a safety net. Let family members and friends help out from time to time!

### Your Safety Net: Family and Friends

Follow these steps to create a "safety net" of people you can rely on during your clinical experience.

1. Explain to your family that your schedule is going to change. Make sure they understand that this opportunity is important and that it's the next big step toward your new career.
2. Tell your family exactly what schedule changes are in store.
3. Offer concrete details about your new schedule.
   - If you have young children, talk with them about when or if they'll be in day care.
   - Talk with your family about which days or nights can be set aside for family time, such as family dinner nights.
   - Give specific jobs, like doing the laundry or helping out with other household chores, to family members who can handle that level of responsibility.
   - Let your family know how much you appreciate their help!
4. Tell your friends about your new schedule, especially those you usually meet with for regularly scheduled events.

5. If you have roommates, make them aware of your schedule changes, especially if you do laundry together, share the cooking or cleaning, or have other commitments.

6. Most importantly, let your family and friends know that they are important to you and this extra demand on your time isn't permanent. You may need their support to help get you through the busy days ahead!

## Embrace Diversity

Chapter 4 describes the many benefits of experiencing diversity in school and society, generally. You will likely also find a great diversity among both the health care professionals and the patients you'll be working with in your clinical experience. This represents another great opportunity to meet a wide range of people and experience many kinds of differences among people. In this way too, your clinical rotation or externship is helping prepare you for your future career in health care.

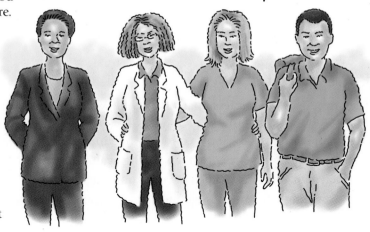

*Life is so much more interesting since we're all different individuals!*

You may want to review the section *What Is Cultural Diversity?* in Chapter 4 before your clinical experience. What is key when working with others different from yourself in some way is to respect them as individuals and remain open-minded. Do not expect everyone to look, dress, act, or think the same as you and your family or friends, but be accepting of differences. The more you interact with others, the more you will understand people with a different background—and the better you will become in your job. Embrace the many differences that contribute so much to our multicultural world.

## PERSONAL AND PROFESSIONAL CODES OF ETHICS

During much of your time at school, you've been focusing on acquiring information, whether that means memorizing key terms, reading about difficult concepts, or figuring out how to apply your new knowledge. There's so much to learn that everything else seems like an unimportant extra. But there's another area that's just as important to your future career in health care—your code of ethics. This becomes particularly important now in your clinical rotation.

In health care, you're often entrusted with intensely personal information about people you don't know. You represent something to the patients you deal with—an ideal of a caring and educated health care professional. You're expected to be trustworthy and to take your job seriously.

You should do everything in your power to live up to this ideal. It may seem impossibly high, but it should be your goal. As you'll see, it's not about being perfect. It's about reminding yourself every day that what you do is not only special, but a privilege and a great responsibility as well.

A professional code of ethics addresses these areas:

- professionalism
- confidentiality
- patient rights and safety
- cultural diversity
- personal conduct

# Professionalism

The first item in the professional code of ethics is professionalism itself. Professionalism means:

- maintaining professional conduct while in the clinical area
- working effectively with others on the health care team
- staying within the bounds of your knowledge and skills
- providing safe care through understanding and following policies and procedures

## PROFESSIONAL AND PERSONAL CONDUCT

Chapter 10 describes what professional and personal conduct means. Remember that patients need to feel that they can trust you to take care of them. Patients will probably see you face to face, whether you're providing direct care or taking their insurance information. They'll size up your character and make decisions about whether you seem to care about them. Similarly, your coworkers need to be reassured that you're capable of carrying out your responsibilities. During your clinical rotation, strive to maintain the same conduct as the health care professionals around you. You're not "just a student" any more.

## GO TEAM!

You might think of your clinical rotation as a time for you to shine by showing how much you've learned and what you can do. And it is. But it's also a time to show that you can be a successful member of a team.

Health care is all about teamwork. For example, an emergency medical technician takes critical vital signs and medical history before handing that information off to the doctor. The doctor makes evaluations based on this information and then orders lab work, x-rays, and medications—all these are accomplished by other team members. Every link in the chain is important. Even if you're in the front office or handling medical billing, your work is critically important to the members of the team providing direct care. By keeping patient records organized and up to date, you help ensure that the health care facility is providing the best care. Likewise, by sending the proper referrals and instructions to the lab, you enable lab personnel to perform necessary tests. And you can protect a patient's safety by informing the pharmacy of any allergies the patient may have to certain drugs.

So, although you should take advantage of every opportunity to shine, remember that being a reliable team member is very valuable.

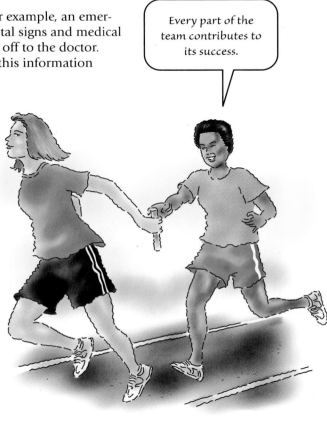

Every part of the team contributes to its success.

## OUT OF BOUNDS

Just as professionalism involves being a team player, knowing the limits of your expertise makes you a trustworthy and professional health care provider.

### There Are No Dumb Questions, Only Dumb Mistakes

There probably will be times when you think you know how to perform a certain task, but you're not completely sure. You may feel reluctant to ask for verification—you might think it makes you look less than knowledgeable. You may be tempted to go with a hunch.

Stop! In health care, you have to be absolutely certain. If you have any questions about what you should do, ask someone who knows.

Don't run the risk of making a mistake with a patient's records, medication, tests, or other procedures. Instead, get the help you need and then carry out the task.

### Know Your Limits

What if your supervisor or another staff person asks you to do something you haven't yet been trained to do? You might be very reluctant to admit that you don't know how to do the task. But this is a situation where you *must* say so. Remember, your clinical rotation is a learning experience. Everyone expects you to need guidance and training. No one expects you to know it all. It is critical that you stay within the bounds of your knowledge and skills.

Also, letting your supervisor and coworkers know your capabilities is vital to keeping the team running properly. Your team will trust you more if they know that you never attempt to do anything unless you're absolutely sure you know how to do it.

## Confidentiality

Patient confidentiality is both an ethical and legal obligation that is just as important for students on clinical rotation as for all health care professionals. Only certain individuals can lawfully receive verbal, written, or electronic patient information. Those who have a need to know patient information include the patient's health care providers and those authorized by the patient to have access to that information. Private patient information is *any* information about a patient, including things, such as:

- health records
- data on billing and payment
- insurance information
- prescriptions
- symptoms and diagnoses
- test results
- personal information unrelated to health care

### KEEPING PATIENT INFORMATION PRIVATE

You might overhear coworkers sharing patient information with each other in a casual way, over lunch, or in the break room. If they encourage you to join in, remember that discussing private patient information is not only unprofessional, it's illegal. So, change the subject or just leave. If you never share information, others will not ask you. This may be difficult, but it's better than getting yourself and your workplace into legal trouble for breaching patient privacy.

## Lips Zipped

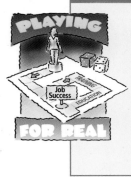

Hi, I'm Donna and I'm training to become a home health aide. I was taking a break with some coworkers one day when they started talking about a couple of patients. They were saying things about the patients' homes and family situations that were very personal. Even though they weren't using the patients' names, I knew this kind of talk was inappropriate. They asked me if I'd been to one of the patient's homes and what I thought about it. I was tempted to get into it, but I knew it wasn't the right thing to do. So I just said, "I don't think we should be talking about this," and changed the subject by asking a question about a homework assignment.

## THE HEALTH INSURANCE PORTABILITY AND ACCOUNTABILITY ACT

The Health Insurance Portability and Accountability Act of 1996, or HIPAA, protects the privacy, confidentiality, and security of all medical records. During your clinical orientation, you'll receive information about maintaining patient rights under HIPAA. The information will be tailored to the health care facility where you're working, as well as your own job tasks. Failure to comply with HIPAA regulations, whether intentional or unintentional, can result in civil penalties. (See *Patient Privacy Rights*.)

## TIPS FOR MAINTAINING PATIENT PRIVACY

Follow these safeguards to help you maintain patient privacy:

- Protect your computer password and log off the computer when you're finished with it. Don't run the risk of an unauthorized person walking by and accessing patient information.
- Keep patient charts closed or put away when not in use.
- Ensure faxes and computer printouts are not left unattended, especially in areas where curious patients are waiting, like the front desk.
- Dispose of unneeded patient information in special receptacles before you leave the facility.
- Do not talk about patients in your casual conversations. This means no conversation about a patient even with the patient's visitors or your family and friends.

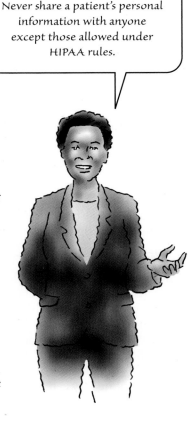

Never share a patient's personal information with anyone except those allowed under HIPAA rules.

- Use a quiet voice when giving necessary information to others on the health care team, whether on the telephone or in person. A listening patient might spread details to other people.
- Remove patient identifying information before handing in written class work.

---

**Patient Privacy Rights**

The goal of HIPAA regulations is to provide safeguards against inappropriate use and release of personal medical information, including all medical records and identifiable health information in any form (electronic, paper, and verbal). HIPAA gives patients the right to:

- give consent before information is released for treatments, payment, or health care operations.
- be educated about the provider's policy on privacy protection.
- access their health records.
- request that their health records be amended for accuracy.
- access the history of nonroutine disclosures (disclosures that didn't occur in the course of treatment, payment, health care operations, or those not specifically authorized by the patient).
- request that the provider restrict the use and routine disclosure of information he or she has. (Providers aren't required to grant this request, especially if they think the information is important to the quality of patient care, such as disclosing HIV status to another medical treatment provider.)

---

# Patient Rights and Safety

Concern for patients' rights and safety should be another part of your professional ethics. You'll not only protect your workplace from legal action, but you'll also be providing the best care to patients. Patients have a number of rights about which you should be aware.

## THE RIGHT TO BE INVOLVED

Patients are more knowledgeable, assertive, and actively involved in their health care than ever before. They analyze their own symptoms and may question their doctors' diagnoses. Some patients even perform home testing before visiting a health care facility. Many patients also demand more information about the risks, alternatives, and benefits associated with the treatment recommended by their doctors. Bills of rights for patients have helped reinforce the public's expectation of quality care. (See *Patient's Bill of Rights*.)

As a member of the health care team, you need to uphold all patient rights as you carry out your duties. Become familiar with your employer's policy on patient rights. View your patients as partners in the health care process and help them get involved in their treatment and care.

## Patient's Bill of Rights

In 1977, the National League for Nursing (NLN) published a patient's bill of rights.

- People have the right to health care that's accessible and that meets professional standards, regardless of where they receive care.
- Patients have the right to courteous and individualized health care that is equitable, humane, and given without discrimination as to race, color, creed, sex, national origin, source of payment, or ethical or political beliefs.
- Patients have the right to information about their diagnosis, prognosis, and treatment, including alternatives to care and risks involved in care, in terms they and their families can easily understand, so they can give informed consent.
- Patients have the legal right to informed participation in all decisions concerning their health care.
- Patients have the right to information about the qualifications, names, and titles of personnel responsible for providing their health care.
- Patients have the right to refuse observation by those not directly involved in their care.
- Patients have the right to privacy during interview, exam, and treatment.
- Patients have the right to privacy in communicating and visiting with persons of their choice.
- Patients have the right to refuse treatments, medications, or participation in research and experimentation, without punitive action being taken against them.
- Patients have the right to coordination and continuity of health care.
- Patients have the right to appropriate instruction or education from health care personnel so they can achieve an optimal level of wellness and an understanding of their basic health needs.

- Patients have the right to confidentiality of all records (except as otherwise provided for by law or third-party payer contracts) and all communications, written or oral, between patients and health care providers.
- Patients have the right of access to all health records pertaining to them, the right to challenge and to have their records corrected for accuracy, and the right to transfer all such records in the case of continuing care.
- Patients have the right to information on the charges for services, including the right to challenge these.
- Above all, patients have the right to be fully informed as to all their rights in all health care settings.

Reprinted with permission from the National League for Nursing. National League for Nursing. (1977). *Nursing's role in patients' rights*. New York: Author.

## KEEP PATIENTS SAFE!

Patient safety is the responsibility of all members of the health care team, including you, whenever you are in the facility. Even if you don't deal with patients in the exam room, you still need to focus on safety. Patient safety is your responsibility whether you see a patient in the front office or in the examination room.

Safety issues vary according to the type of facility and the capabilities and needs of individual patients. You can, however, take basic steps to reduce each patient's risk.

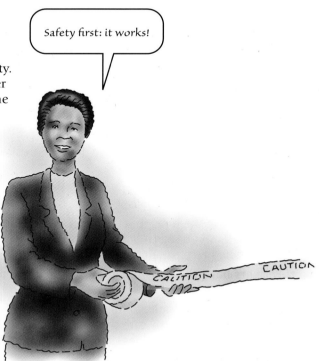

*Safety first: it works!*

### Trip and Fall Hazards

Falls can be caused by many factors: medication, debris on the floor, or out-of-place equipment. So be vigilant and protective of your patients. Even if you feel that your work area is well out of range for patient falls, remember that patients travel through most parts of a facility. As the receptionist, for example, you would want to check the waiting area periodically to make sure there are no magazines on the floor, tables too close to chairs, or large potted plants too close to seats; all of these are potential trip-and-fall hazards. Or as a medical assistant walking down a hallway in a patient treatment area, for example, you would be alert for a wet spot that makes a floor slippery or an electrical cord over which a patient could trip; such conditions should be immediately reported or corrected.

### Equipment Safety

You're responsible for making sure that the equipment you have been trained and authorized to use for patient care is free from defects. You're also responsible for using that equipment properly and following instructions in the procedure manual. If you have questions about equipment use, ask your supervisor or instructor.

### Prevent Disease Transmission

To reduce the risk of transmitting disease, wash your hands frequently! Proper hand washing (with soap and water or waterless soap) is the single most effective thing you can do to prevent the spread of infection. Follow guidelines for washing between patients, wearing gloves at appropriate times, and following other facility policies for preventing disease transmission.

### PROTECT YOURSELF!

While providing safe care for patients, you also must protect yourself. Prevention is the key to keeping yourself safe in the workplace.

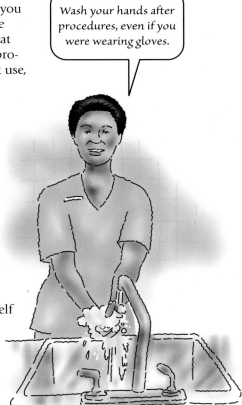

*Wash your hands after procedures, even if you were wearing gloves.*

### Infection: The Buck Stops Here

To protect yourself from infection, you should handle the following as if they contain infectious organisms:

- all blood and other body fluids
- human tissue
- mucous membranes
- broken skin

This means you should follow standard precautions at all times. For example, you must wear gloves for procedures that might expose you to a patient's blood or other body fluids. (See *Stop the Spread of Infection.*) Even if a patient appears healthy, the same precautions always apply.

## Stop the Spread of Infection

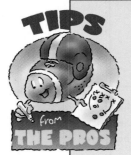

The Centers for Disease Control and Prevention (CDC) publishes guidelines to provide the widest possible protection against the transmission of infection. CDC officials recommend that health care workers handle all blood and other body fluids, tissues, mucous membranes, and broken skin as if they contained infectious agents, regardless of the patient's diagnosis, and to take the following precautions:

- Wash your hands before and after patient care, after removing gloves, or immediately after contamination with blood, body fluids, excretions, secretions, or drainage.
- Wear gloves if you will or might come in contact with blood or other body fluids, specimens, tissues, secretions, excretions, mucous membranes, broken skin, or contaminated objects or surfaces.
- Change gloves and wash your hands between patients. When caring for the same patient, change gloves and wash your hands if you touch anything with a high concentration of microorganisms.
- Wear a fluid-resistant gown, eye protection, and a mask during procedures that are likely to generate droplets of blood or bodily fluids.
- Carefully handle used patient care equipment that's soiled with blood or body fluids; follow facility guidelines for cleaning and disinfecting equipment and environmental surfaces.
- Keep contaminated linens away from your body and place in properly labeled containers.
- Handle needles and sharps carefully and immediately discard them in a designated disposal unit after use; use sharps with safety features whenever possible.
- Immediately notify your supervisor of a needlestick or sharp instrument injury, mucosal splash, or contamination of nonintact skin with blood or other body fluids to initiate appropriate investigation of the incident and care.
- Use mouthpieces, resuscitation bags, or ventilation devices in place of mouth-to-mouth resuscitation.
- If occupational exposure to blood is likely, you should be vaccinated against hepatitis B.
- Become familiar with your facility's infection control policies and procedures.

## When Accidents Happen...

If you are injured by a sharp instrument, or if any of your mucous membranes are contacted by blood or other body fluids, notify your clinical instructor or supervisor immediately. This person will:

- help you with immediate first aid
- fill out an accident report
- ensure that you receive the proper follow-up care

Depending on your duties during your clinical rotation, you may be at risk of occupational exposure to hepatitis B. If so, your school might require you to get the hepatitis B vaccine series.

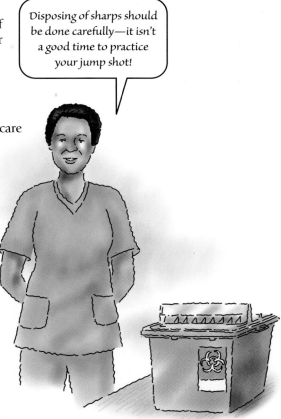

*Disposing of sharps should be done carefully—it isn't a good time to practice your jump shot!*

## Be Kind to Your Back

Back injuries are common among health care employees. Many patient care facilities and laboratories require you to push, pull, lift, and carry heavy objects or equipment. People working in records or billing may have to move boxes of files. By using proper body mechanics, you can avoid back injuries:

- Keep a low center of gravity by flexing your hips and knees instead of bending at the waist. This position distributes weight evenly between your upper and lower body and helps maintain balance.

- Create a wide base of support by spreading your feet apart. This tactic provides lateral stability and lowers your body's center of gravity.

- Maintain proper body alignment and keep your body's center of gravity directly over the base of support by moving your feet rather than twisting and bending at the waist.

## Handle Chemicals With Care

Many potentially hazardous chemicals are used in health care facilities. Certain drugs, powerful cleaning solutions, and disinfectants are common hazards. A material safety data sheet (MSDS) provides you with information about the physical and chemical hazards that can occur from these substances. Each MSDS provides information about the chemicals found in a substance and how to treat exposure to that substance. Every health care facility has an MSDS manual. Make sure you know where the manual is located in your facility. Tell your clinical instructor immediately if you are exposed to any potentially hazardous chemical.

# PLANNING AHEAD

As you look forward to your upcoming clinical rotation, there are some ways you can prepare so you hit the ground running on your first day:

- Know the dress code.
- Know the equipment.
- Know your mentor.
- Know the clinic.

## Suit Up

Professionalism starts with something that might seem trivial: clothes. Just as athletes have to suit up before a game, you'll need to dress appropriately for *your* big game—your clinical experience. You might be thinking that just wearing a uniform ensures you're dressing correctly. Not true! Yes, you probably will be wearing a uniform (e.g., scrubs). But there are other important points to keep in mind to make sure you're dressed appropriately.

> "Suiting up" for your clinical rotation means dressing like a true health care professional. Check with your clinical mentor if you have any questions about dress.

- Keep your uniform clean. This can be hard to do in a clinical setting, but it's important. A stained or wrinkled uniform tells patients and staff members that you don't take your work seriously.
- Wear your identification badge pinned near your collarbone. Clipping it lower such as near your waist makes it less visible to people who need to see who you are.
- Choose professional shoes of a style worn by professionals in the facility's department. Don't wear sneakers, sandals, or clogs unless you know for sure that they're allowed where you'll be working.

Aside from your uniform, there is another dress factor to keep in mind: keep it simple. Many people are tempted to wear jewelry, perfume or cologne, or an unusual hairstyle. But when you're at work, you shouldn't try to stand out with an original look. You should stand out because of your excellent skills and positive attitude. Professionals don't call attention to their looks on the job. They let their skills do the talking.

Some health care facilities have stricter guidelines about dress than others. Ask any questions you may have about dress code during your clinical orientation. Your clinical mentor or instructor will give you specific guidelines to follow. If you're ever unsure as to whether a particular item of clothing or accessory is appropriate, play it safe until you've checked with your instructor.

## Know the Equipment

You will be given a list of equipment you'll need for your clinical rotation. Make sure you have all the necessary supplies with you on your first day. You should also bring:

- a notebook
- a pen or pencil
- personal identification (such as a Social Security card, driver's license, or student ID)

These additional items will come in handy in case you need to fill out any paperwork on your first day. You may need proof of identification to obtain a parking permit or an identification badge. If you drive to the facility, write down your car's license plate number in your notebook; you might need to register your car with the facility if you park in a garage.

Another helpful piece of equipment is a personal data assistant (PDA). Software for a PDA can take the place of a drug book, textbook, and other references. A PDA, like many cell phones, also may have functions that can simplify your life, such as a calculator, address book, calendar, to-do list, and memo pad.

As a general rule, it's best to leave your cell phone turned off completely during work hours. Professionals do not allow themselves to be distracted by outside calls while on the job and patients and other health care workers will be irritated if you take a call on the job or are even seen checking for messages while working. Use your cell phone only on your personal break time. If you must leave the phone on to receive a call in case of an emergency, such as a call from your child's school or day care provider, then set it to vibrate rather than ring and keep it in your pocket.

## Know Your Mentor

Your clinical mentor (or preceptor) will coach you through your clinical experience. Do your best to start out on the right foot with your mentor—you just might learn something! Also, try to avoid making judgments about your mentor based on what you may have heard from other students. Remember that professionals interact with a wide range of other people without being influenced by personal opinions.

### NO NAME GAMES

Remember to be polite and respectful. Address your mentor as Mr., Mrs., Dr., Ms., or by a first name, according to your mentor's stated preference. It's part of the mutual respect you want in your relationship.

## BACKGROUND CHECK

If appropriate, it may be useful to learn a little about how your mentor reached his or her present position. For instance, you might ask questions about how they got into health care, where they went to school, and the positions they have held. But don't pry or overwhelm them with questions. These topics are general enough to come up in conversation.

You should have regular conversations with your mentor about what you're learning and doing. He or she will be happy to answer your questions and to see that you're eager to learn.

## HEAD OFF TROUBLE

If you feel you're unable to develop a good relationship with your mentor, make an appointment to discuss your concerns. If you can't resolve the problems together, follow the procedures outlined in your student handbook for resolving problems.

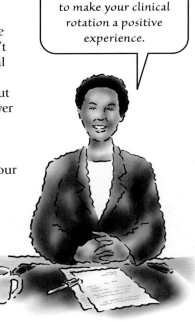

Work with your mentor to make your clinical rotation a positive experience.

## Know the Facility

Because every health care facility is unique in some ways, you should enter your experience there with an open mind, ready to learn. Make an effort from the start to learn how the particular facility does things so you can fit in with the team as soon as possible. Important first steps include:

1. Attend your clinical orientation.
2. Work out the logistics before your first day.
3. Know the policies and rules.
4. Have a good attitude.

## CLINICAL ORIENTATION

Clinical orientation usually takes place at the facility where you'll be doing your rotation. It typically includes a welcome from a representative of the facility, followed by information about the facility. In addition to specifics about what you'll be doing, you may learn:

- the facility's mission statement
- fire and safety procedures
- confidentiality rules

If you will be working with a computer, your orientation may also include computer classes and password assignment.

Your mentor will explain the expectations for your rotation. You'll receive a schedule along with any written assignments and due dates. Clinical objectives and evaluation procedures also will be reviewed at this time, so be sure to ask questions if you have them.

## LOGISTICS

You'll need to consider lots of smaller details before you begin your clinical experience. Where should you park? Whom do you call if you're sick or will be late? Do you need to wear a pager if you leave the facility for lunch?

Remember to ask these types of questions during orientation. The last thing you want at the end of your first day is to find that your car has been towed. Or to hear one day that your supervisor did not learn that you had called in sick until the day was half over. And you don't want to come back from lunch to find out that everyone has been frantically looking for you!

*Make sure you get to work on time—take traffic and parking into consideration.*

## READ THE RULE BOOK

In health care, it's important to do things by the book. Facilities have policies and procedures for virtually every task, from filing to phlebotomy. These rules help ensure that everyone in the facility does things the same way, preventing errors or confusion about what was done or how it was done.

To prepare for your clinical experience, get a copy of the policy and procedures manual ahead of time so you can study it. When you're on the job, know where the manual is stored and refer to it before trying something new. You must always follow a facility's procedures, even if they are slightly different from what you learned in school.

Sometimes a policy or procedure may seem tedious, yet you must still follow it to the letter every time. One major reason for this is safety. Following procedures means you will be doing things correctly. If a patient develops a problem, you'll know that you didn't contribute to it. You can confidently report to your supervisors that you performed your tasks accurately. You'll be ready to enter your career as a professional.

## ATTITUDE—THE LAST WORD

This should be obvious but sometimes isn't: just because you are in the facility for clinical rotation or an externship rather than working a "real job" there, this doesn't mean you shouldn't take it very seriously. You are there working, but you're also there to learn. The facility doesn't *have* to invite you in and provide this valuable experience for you. In other words, be aware that as a student in a clinical rotation, you are a guest in the facility. Be sure you act like a good guest, behaving in a way that will lead to your being invited back.

## CHAPTER SUMMARY

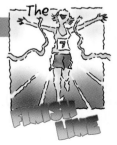

- Because a clinical rotation or externship is a professional experience, practice good personal and professional conduct.
- Protect patients' rights by familiarizing yourself with the Patient's Bill of Rights.
- Guard patient privacy by following HIPAA rules.
- Work to ensure safety for all patients while also protecting yourself.
- Learn about your facility's safety rules by reading the policy and procedures manual.
- Plan for a successful clinical experience. Dress appropriately, bring the right books and supplies, and make sure you arrive on time!

## REVIEW QUESTIONS

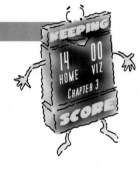

1. How can you practice skills in a clinical setting before your rotation begins?
2. Why is it important to know your limits when you're working in health care?
3. Describe a mentor's role in your clinical experience.
4. List key steps to take in preparation for beginning your clinical experience.
5. Describe the importance of teamwork for the activities you will be engaged in during your clinical rotation.

## CHAPTER ACTIVITIES

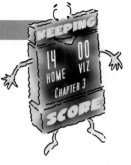

1. Calm Your Fears: Make a list of any aspects of your upcoming clinical experience that you are concerned about. Then write down questions to ask your instructor that will help you better understand and prepare for these things.
2. Act It Out: Get together with three to five classmates. Each of you should write down the steps of a task or a clinical procedure you will perform during the clinical rotation. Then practice or act out each procedure or task until everyone in the group feels comfortable with the steps and ready for the clinical experience.

## CHAPTER 12

# Succeeding in Your Future

WINNING STRATEGY

**WINNING STRATEGY**

*On completion of this chapter and the learning activities you will be able to:*

- See your dreams becoming reality
- Understand the positive choices you make each day
- Explain how to carry your new skills and knowledge into the future
- Know what's involved in the job application process and how to find and get the position you've been dreaming of

You're likely finishing reading this book while still near the beginning of your academic program, but it's still worthwhile to take a look at where you're headed in the future. This chapter will help you connect what you are learning now, and what you have learned in this book, with your future career in health care. You'll also get a head start with information about the job application process you'll be going through as you enter your career. Though this may seem off in the future, understanding the process has great value in the here and now.

## BUILDING ON YOUR ACCOMPLISHMENTS

Now that you're nearing the end of this book, it's a good time to look back on what brought you to this point. Are you closer to fulfilling your original dreams? What obstacles have you overcome along the way? What goals have you accomplished? And most important for this chapter, what skills and knowledge will you be able to use in the future?

You've come a long way since you first opened this book. You've learned how to:

- set and meet goals
- plan ahead and be prepared
- schedule multiple activities and meet deadlines
- identify and deal with stress and anxiety
- listen effectively and apply your critical thinking skills
- meet the challenges of learning and take responsibility for the results
- network and contribute in group activities
- explore optional resources to help you get ahead
- meet standards of professionalism and uphold patients' rights

Now imagine yourself 5 or 10 years down the road, working in your chosen career. Look back at the list above of all of the things that you have already learned. You can apply every one of these new skills to help you succeed in all of your future career and education goals. Ask any health care professional and they'll readily agree, for example, that being able to schedule multiple activities and plan ahead are critical to their job success.

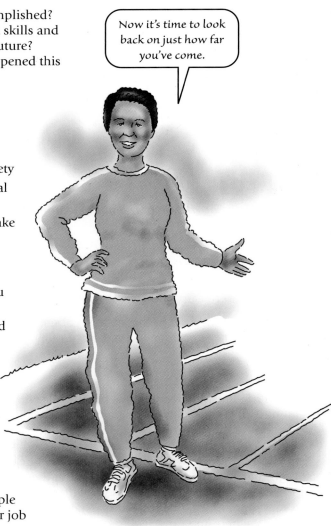

## Make Your Dream a Reality

Even if you're still a year or more away from starting your career in health care, you have done the hardest, most important part: taking action. You tackled the sometimes difficult and complicated task of applying to school and enrolling in courses. You shuffled your work and other responsibilities to make time for class. You studied hard and completed your coursework. All these things have brought you closer to making your dream a reality.

It's important to recognize and take pride in your accomplishments, no matter how small they may seem at the time. Celebrate each success now, whether it's doing well on a test, completing a research project, or forming a study group with a few fellow students. Remember, it's the small steps that move you toward accomplishing big things!

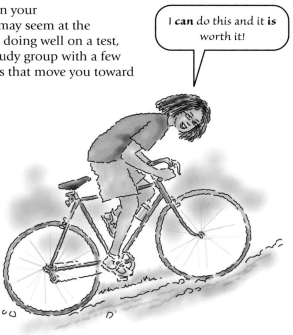

I **can** do this and it **is** worth it!

## Courage

You've also shown to yourself and proved to those around you that you have the courage and fortitude to stick with it and meet your goals. It takes courage to believe in yourself and to believe that you can make changes in terms of your education and future career. It takes courage to say, "I *can* do this and it *is* worth it." Carry that attitude through your transition into the professional world of work.

### Having the Courage to Succeed

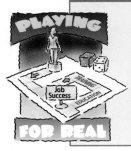

My name is Leila. When I first thought about starting school, I was intimidated. It was a big financial and emotional investment for my family and me. What if I couldn't handle it and had to drop out after one semester? I was worried about what people would think. But then I remembered how my uncle always used to say, "Nothing ventured, nothing gained." If I never took a chance, I'd never achieve anything. I decided it was better to take a chance than to tell myself I couldn't do it.

## Choices

To make it this far, you had to have faith in your choices. You've had to make many decisions about your education, your courses, and your career goals. In so doing, you've improved your decision-making skills, which will remain important as you move into your career.

As you approach the end of your educational program, you'll face many new decisions as you look for the career position that best meets your needs and desires. You'll have to decide where to look for a job, perhaps what specific kind of job to pursue, and how to apply and interview most successfully. This chapter introduces that process and will help you get started.

Touchdown! Every time you overcome an obstacle to your success, take time to celebrate!

## MEETING CHALLENGES

You know it hasn't been easy to arrive at where you are today. By the time you complete your educational program, you will have overcome many obstacles, likely including financing your education, finding time for studying and the rest of your life, and managing relationships and family life through a long, stressful period.

How have you overcome these obstacles to your success? You've learned may techniques in this book already, including ways to cope with stress, build confidence, and accept the support of others.

In your future career, you similarly will face new challenges. Things change fast in health care and your job undoubtedly will also change. You will be given new responsibilities and you'll be asked to do more. As technology advances, you'll need to learn new knowledge and skills. But your experience now as a student will have prepared you well to meet those challenges, too.

## GO-O-O-AL!

When you think of your main goal as a student, you probably see yourself working in your new health care career. But you also have many smaller goals between now and that future:

- doing well in your courses
- learning new skills
- finding the right job

These are big picture goals you'll reach by achieving smaller goals, such as keeping your study schedule, attending class, balancing work and school, and registering for the right courses—all the things we've been talking about throughout this book.

> *Adjust your short-term goals to make sure you reach your long-term go-o-o-al!*

## Your Goals and You: A Long-Term Relationship

As you look ahead to the future, review the goals you were asked to think about at the beginning of this book. Remember there are four categories of goals:

- *Long-term.* These are things you hope to accomplish in the next 5 to 10 years.
- *Intermediate.* These are things you would like to accomplish in the next 3 to 5 years.
- *Short-term.* These goals are 6 months to 2 years into the future.
- *Immediate.* These are things you hope to accomplish today, this week, or this month.

Remember too that your goals need to be realistic, measurable, and reachable.

## Change Can Be Good

Students adjust their goals for many reasons. Maybe they found their original goals to be unrealistic once they actually started school. Maybe as they began taking courses, they became interested in a different career. These are good reasons to adjust your goals. As you review your goals, ask yourself the following questions:

- Have any of my goals changed since I started school? If so, how and why have they changed?

**How Are You Doing?**

Take some time to evaluate your progress so far by writing your goals here.

Long-Term Goal:

1. _____

Intermediate Goals:

1. _____

2. _____

Short-Term Goals:

1. _____

2. _____

3. _____

Immediate Goals:

1. _____

2. _____

3. _____

Now, ask yourself these questions:

1. When I started reading this book, what immediate or short-term goals had I hoped to accomplish by now? Have I accomplished these goals?

2. If there are goals I have not accomplished, what stopped me?

3. How did I accomplish my other goals?

4. What can I do differently next term to make sure I meet all my immediate or short-term goals?

5. What are two or three new immediate goals I can accomplish today, this week, or this month?

- How do I feel when I make adjustments to my goals? Is it discouraging (I feel like I failed to meet my original goals) or empowering (I know I can adjust my goals without giving up on them)?

Remember, it's always better to modify your goals or your time line than to give up!

When you choose to adjust your goals, avoid seeing changes as a failure of any sort. Instead, be happy with your new goals and focus on finding creative ways to keep moving forward. Being flexible is critical to your success.

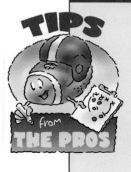

## Adjusting Your Goals

If you feel uncomfortable about changing your goals, talk to an academic advisor or someone else you trust.

1. Tell your advisor what adjustments you're considering.
2. Give your reasons for considering the adjustments.
3. Ask your advisor if your adjustments seem positive or whether there may be a way to continue working toward your original goals.

If you talk to someone who is encouraging and supportive, you can feel at ease listening to that person's advice. But in the end, only you can decide if you really need to change your goals.

## A Rewarding Experience

To many students, graduation day is when you're rewarded for all your hard work. Others may see the first day of their new career as the big reward. But those long-term benefits may still be far away in the future.

That's why you should give yourself small rewards along the way. If you do well on a big test, for example, maybe you could go out with friends to celebrate. If you finish a big project you've been working on for weeks, consider taking a Saturday off to do something fun. The kinds of rewards are up to you. The point is to reward yourself for all of your achievements, big and small, so you can stay motivated to keep going!

## CARRYING YOUR NEW SKILLS INTO THE FUTURE

You're on the track to success as a student and in your career. You've learned a lot about what it takes to do well in school. Five or 10 years from now, these things will be just as important. Here are just a few of the characteristics and skills you've been developing that will continue to be important in your future career:

- *Motivation.* Whether motivated by an intrinsic desire to succeed or a curiosity to learn new things, or extrinsic motivators such as good grades or a higher paying job down the road, your motivation to complete your education should carry over into your career. In the same way, you will be motivated to do your job well, and in the same way you will find success! Motivation is the key to overcome obstacles both in school and on the job.

- *Positive attitude.* If you believe you can do something, you'll find a way to do it. Believing in yourself—having a positive attitude—is the first step toward accomplishing your goals. A positive attitude helps you identify and accept your responsibilities in the learning process and on the job. This has already helped you study effectively and continually improve your grades. In the future, your positive attitude will continue to help you advance in your career. In addition, everyone enjoys working with a person who is a pleasure to be around!

- *Persistence.* Doing your best even during difficult times is a very important life skill. In all health care settings, there are difficult times. For example, during cold and flu season demands on your time may be greater and your work days more hectic. Everyone has tough times; it's how you respond to them that matters.

- *Learning abilities.* Learning how to study well for your courses will likely be more valuable than you can guess once you are in your new career—and not just because you will continue to learn new things on the job. You're also learning now how to stay focused. Working through distractions is a critical skill, whether you're in class or in the middle of a task at work. Health care is a very busy business! Your ability to focus and stay on task will be put to the test daily.

- *Managing stress and taking care of yourself.* You've come to realize stress is a part of life and especially life as a student. It would be nice to think you'll never feel stressed again after graduation, but that's just a pleasant day dream! Remember to keep practicing ways to reduce the stress you feel, including maintaining your physical and mental health, and these good habits will carry into your future job as well. Although there will always be stressful situations, you don't have to feel stressed out when you've developed ways to cope and succeed!

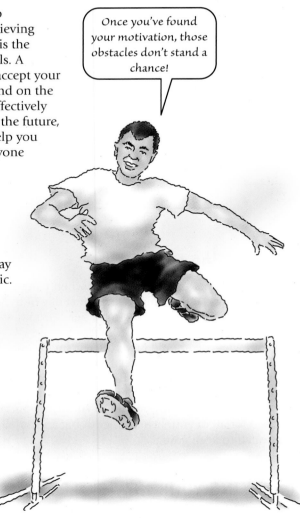

Once you've found your motivation, those obstacles don't stand a chance!

- *Managing your time and resources.* In school, you have to plan for study time, class time, tests, and so much more to accomplish everything. You've already learned a lot about time management and these skills will carry over into work as well. For example, you'll need to create a schedule that allows you to get everything done efficiently and accurately. You'll likely also have to manage resources in the same way you're now managing your financial life as a student.

- *Interacting with others.* You've already learned much about how to interact successfully with your instructors and other students and you will continue to refine these networking and communication skills. At school, other students can be valuable sources of information and support. Your network will also be valuable when you are conducting your first job search. Then, at work, coworkers can offer the same benefits.

- *Speaking the language.* You may feel like a rookie in your first semester or term at school, but you already know much more than you did before. You've begun to "speak the language" by picking up new knowledge and skills related to your future career. As a professional, you'll continue to gain more knowledge and learn new techniques. In addition, you've learned much about the career you've chosen. Knowing what to expect helps you make informed decisions for your future. Keep reminding yourself that you've come a long way so far; you owe it to yourself to keep going!

- *Knowing your way around.* In school, you're doing more than simply reading textbooks and going to class. You might be networking with classmates, learning to manage a busy schedule, and using available campus resources. These accomplishments can increase your confidence, which will help you get the job done in your future career. Becoming an expert at school will make it easier to become an expert in the work-place. You'll be ahead of the game when it's easy for you to learn where everything is kept, who can help you solve problems, and how to get information quickly.

> Stretch yourself to become an even more active learner!

## Shake It Off!

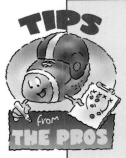

*TIPS from THE PROS*

When you get nervous about the obstacles you face, you can become fearful of them. This leads you to doubt your ability to overcome those obstacles, which might make you discouraged. Taking small steps can help you shake off those feelings of fear, doubt, and discouragement.

For example, one of the biggest challenges you may have faced is learning how to be an active learner. When you're working and going to class, as well as fulfilling other responsibilities, you may not have a lot of energy left to ask questions in class, visit your instructor during office hours, join a study group, take on an internship, or go the extra mile to get your education.

> You're not a rookie anymore—even if you've just started school, you've already learned a lot!

But as you took each of these small steps, it probably became easier to extend yourself. Now that you're in the habit of being an active learner, it's become second nature. And there are other things you can do to become an even more active learner. If you joined a study group, why not lead one? If you know what field you want to enter, why not set up some informational interviews with professionals working in that field? It's just a matter of taking what you're already doing one step further.

And being an active learner now is good practice for being a go-getter on the job. Everyone knows that the go-getters do better in their chosen careers. Think about it. If you had to hire someone to get things done, would you choose the applicant who waited to be told what to do?

## Getting Comfortable With People

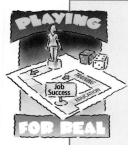

I'm Thomas. I've always been a quiet person and when I first started college, I was kind of shy. I didn't go out of my way to meet new people or strike up conversations. But I was invited to join a study group with other students I didn't know and gradually I opened up more. It took a while, but by the end of my program I'd gotten comfortable introducing myself to strangers and talking with new people. And when I started my first job as a medical assistant, was I ever happy I'd developed some skills interacting with others. In our clinic, I greet the patients, bring them back to the exam room, and ask questions about their health issues. If I'd started this job being as shy as I was when I started college, I might have disappeared at lunch time and never gone back! But, instead, I've learned how to interact comfortably with all kinds of people and I really enjoy my work at the clinic.

# GETTING YOUR FIRST PROFESSIONAL JOB

Soon you'll be looking for your first full-time job in health care or a part-time or summer job for experience. You'll need a well-written résumé, an eye-catching cover letter, and polished interviewing skills. But where do you begin? Just as when you started school, the first step is the hardest. Here are some pointers to get you to the next step.

## Learning the Ropes

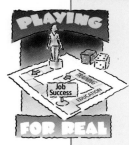

I'm Charles. When I first started school, I was really lost. The campus seemed huge. Every time I needed to do something, like sign up for courses or ask about my financial aid, I was told to go to some building I'd never heard of. My instructors all had materials on reserve at the library and I wasn't sure how to get them. And I was embarrassed to ask questions all the time. I thought it made me look dumb.

But there was no way around it, so I had to swallow my pride and ask. And you know what? I found out that people were happy to help me. No one thought I was dumb. After a few weeks, I didn't have the same problems any more—I knew where things were. Then *I* could be the one to help other students, which made me feel confident—like a leader. I realized that finding my way around campus wasn't an impossible challenge; it was just part of the learning process.

## Writing Your Résumé

Students often seek the "perfect" résumé format to guarantee they'll get the job they want, but in reality there is no one correct or best way to write a résumé. You can spend some time on websites that present a variety of résumé formats, to get ideas about what organization and appearance best fits your own experience, background, and personality.

One more word about résumé appearance. Increasingly, job applications are being submitted online. The facility's website, for example, may ask you to submit your résumé by copying it into an online form. Often, this means that special formatting you may have worked on so hard to make your résumé look great on paper is lost when you cut and paste into their form. It can be reduced to a "plain text" version without boldface, italics, large fonts, bullet points, etc. What this really means is that they're much more inter-ested in the substance of the résumé than what it looks like. What does it actually say about you?

Remember also that a résumé doesn't actually get you the job—its goal is to get you an interview. An employer who posts a job opening may receive dozens of résumés. You can't guess all the precise characteristics the employer is looking for, but your résumé can show what you yourself are like. If you are a match, then you're more likely to reach the interview stage.

New graduates often worry that they have less chance of being the one an employer is interested in and this lack of confidence can lead to an uninspiring résumé. But that's not how you should be thinking! For example, if like most new graduates you haven't yet worked in the career position you're seeking, you may worry that the job will go to someone with more experience. Actually, however, if it is an entry-level position, the employer may specifically be seeking someone without direct experience—and someone who has already worked for years in the field can be at a disadvantage for that job. The employer may want you to be open and flexible and willing to learn how things are done at

> Learning the ropes will help you become more confident. And when you're working in health care, it's very important to be confident in your abilities!

their particular health care facility and, as a new graduate, you may be perfect. You might land a job because in the past, even as a part-time student job, you developed certain skills—such as working with a variety of people, or handling money, or working on a computer, or working with math, or anything else you may have done—that the employer is seeking for this specific position. You really can't know *exactly* what they want, but you can honestly present your strengths, whatever they are, so that the employer can see how you may be right for the job. So don't worry about competing for jobs with others who have more experience, or different experience. You'll get the job where they want *you*—they just need to see who you are! That's what your résumé will do for you in this process.

Regardless of format, every résumé is built on the same basics:

- contact information—your name, phone number(s), address, and email address
- education—relevant courses you've completed, diplomas, certifications, or degrees you've earned, along with educational honors and achievements
- work experience—relevant positions you have held, along with your responsibilities and achievements in them, and the names and addresses of your past employers and the dates you worked for them

In addition, you should consider including:

- your objective—the title of the job position you want or one or two sentences about what you want to do
- skills, traits, and achievements relevant to the job—for example, computer skills, language skills, people skills, technical skills (be specific! Don't just say "proficient with computers" but list types of programs you're good at)
- references—contact information for former employers who have been impressed with your work (only if there is room without your résumé becoming too long)

If you don't put references on your résumé, have a separate list available for any interviewer who requests it.

In general, a good résumé is easy to read and neat (no coffee stains!), has no typos or spelling errors (proofread twice!), and shows a potential employer why you are the person for the job without exaggerating your abilities. See *Characteristics of a Good Résumé.*

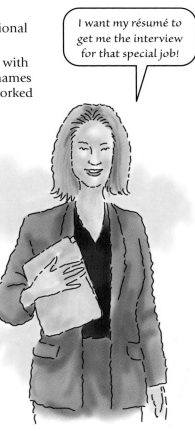

I want my résumé to get me the interview for that special job!

### Characteristics of a Good Résumé

- A short résumé is better than a long one. One page is enough unless if you have a lot of relevant experience.

- Focus on what you've actually done, not just position titles. Use strong verbs (e.g., *analyzed, chaired, created, developed, implemented, managed, organized, performed, planned, researched, wrote,* etc.).

- Use specific numbers when appropriate to describe what you accomplished at work and in school. If you're proud of your GPA, for example, include it.

- Use keywords related to the specific job or career. Some hiring managers review submitted résumés with software that looks for keywords.

- Be sure information is easy to find. Use the standard convention of using a reverse chronological listing of experience, starting with your current or most recent job and moving backward in time, unless you have a good reason for using a different format.

- Unless the position you are applying for is almost always identical in all health care facilities, customize your résumé for the specific application rather than sending one "generic" résumé everywhere. For example, if an advertised position mentions they're looking for applicants with "people skills," make sure the résumé you submit has some specifics about working with people—not just a listing of your technical skills.

- With paper résumés, follow conventional appearance. Do not use a font size smaller than 11 points. Use 1-inch margins all the way around. Print your résumé on a quality bright white paper.

## Finding Openings

As you're working on your résumé, you should also be starting your search for job openings for which you may apply. There are many different ways you can find out about open positions. If you look only in the want ads, you'd likely not discover many positions for which you are qualified. Successful job applicants consider every possible avenue in their job search:

- Listings in your school's placement or career office
- Online listings on job bulletin boards (do an Internet search for "*career title* jobs")

- Listings with professional associations or in professional journals or websites
- Classified ads (newspapers, Craigslist.com)
- Word of mouth (check with everyone in your network)
- Websites of health care facilities

## Composing a Cover Letter

You should always include a cover letter with every résumé you send out. This will improve the odds that your résumé will get the attention it deserves. In fact, the whole purpose of a cover letter is to motivate the reader to look carefully at your résumé.

A good cover letter is not, however, your résumé in paragraph form. Instead, use the cover letter to tell more about yourself and why you want that particular job—and most important, why you would be good at it. Write a separate, individualized cover letter for each employer to whom you are sending your résumé. Carefully study the job description and analyze what they're looking for. What are the key words they use in the description? Talk to friends or others knowledgeable about the type of work or the specific facility, if possible, and ask what kind of people work there and what the "climate" is like. Then review your own interests and background for specifics that will suggest how you'll fit in perfectly.

Be sure to address the cover letter to the specific person or company to which you are applying. Keep in mind also that your cover letter shows how well you communicate, which is important in many careers. Write clearly—and carefully! You're making a first impression with your cover letter and you won't get a second chance if you misspell the name of the facility or use sloppy grammar and punctuation. After you polish the letter to your best, ask someone to read it, whose judgment you trust and who won't just automatically tell you it's great.

As with your résumé, keep the formatting simple because you may have to cut and paste it into an online form.

Finally, don't be discouraged if you never hear back after making an application or receive only a form letter response. Long gone are the days when companies used to respond individually to every job applicant; many companies no longer respond at all to applicants who are not invited to an interview. Remember that there may have been many, many applicants—and that they are not rejecting you personally. It just means they aren't perfect match for you. Don't let it affect your self-confidence. After all, now you're free to find and accept a job that *is* a perfect match with your interests and skills!

## Acing the Interview

Your résumé and cover letter get you the interview, but they don't get you the job. For many students, this is where the real stress of the job application process sets in. Remember to use the stress reduction techniques described in earlier chapters!

Think of your interview as your first day on the job. But it is also like the first day of your clinical rotation and you will have already been through that. So you should have the confidence you need to give a good interview even if you're nervous. Remember: *all* job applicants are nervous and the person interviewing you knows and accepts that.

Here are some guidelines for the interview:

Do:

- Be on time! Check the address and directions ahead of time, know where to park if you're driving, know how long it will take to get to the building at that time of day, and give yourself a little extra time to collect your thoughts as you walk to the office.
- Wear serious, modest clothing and look professional and competent.
- Bring a notebook and pen, in addition to extra copies of your résumé and list of references.
- Make pleasant eye contact, shake hands with confidence, and remember your interviewer's name.
- Ask questions. After all, you're trying to decide whether to work for them as much as they're trying to decide whether to hire you. Questions also demonstrate your interest and motivation.

Did you notice that everything in this list sounds familiar? That's because you've learned about all of these things in previous chapters on being a successful student. Now you're simply applying them in another setting!

Don't:

- Eat, drink, chew gum, wear headphones, or let your cell phone ring.
- Flirt or promise anything you can't deliver.
- Exaggerate (or lie!) about anything in your background. Anything later discovered or perceived to be a falsehood is grounds for immediate dismissal.

Although you can't exactly practice an interview with someone you already know, you can rehearse what you will say to certain kinds of questions you should expect in an interview. Think about what you will say to questions such as these:

- Tell me about yourself.
- Why did you choose to enter this career field?
- Why do you want to work here more than somewhere else?
- Why should we hire you?
- Where do you see yourself in 5 years? In 10 years?
- What are your primary strengths?
- What are your weaknesses?

New applicants can be thrown off by that last question—after all, you're ready to talk about your experiences and skills and suddenly they're asking what you are *not* good at! In part, this question is designed to test your honesty. Everyone has some weakness and a job applicant who brags that there's really nothing he or she isn't good at will seem arrogant and not make a very good impression. The key here is to turn a negative into a positive. For example, if you feel your math skills are weak, you could admit that (especially if math is not a big part of the job you're applying for), and then go on to say that because you never felt strong in math, you've learned to work hard at it and now you always check your work twice to guard against mistakes. You've turned a weakness into a strength!

The bottom line is that your résumé, cover letter, and interview should be honest and confident. Don't oversell yourself, but don't sell yourself short either.

## Following Up the Interview

Immediately after the interview, write some notes for yourself about what you learned in the interview. You may have new questions now about the job or the work environment, which you'll want to ask if you are invited back. In some cases, employers have a second interview in more depth; if invited back for a second interview, you'll want to be ready to discuss things the first interviewer indicated are important or emphasized in their questions.

Within a day after the interview, send a short thank you note to each person you interviewed with. Try to make this message significant by referring to something in the interview that made an impression on you. You might say, for example, how much you enjoyed learning about the facility and that now you are even more interested in working there because of . . . . You can send your thank you note by email if you have the interviewer's email address, especially if your communication with the employer has been online.

Then there's nothing you can do but wait for a response. In the meantime, continue to look for other openings and make additional applications. And, more than anything, don't get discouraged if you don't get the job. As with your original application, this only means that you and the employer aren't a perfect match—not that they found anything wrong with you personally. So keep looking until you find that perfect match where the best career position awaits!

## A PARTING WORD

You've reached the end of this book and, although you're likely to still have some time from reaching the end of your academic program, you're better prepared now for the rest of your education and entry into your career thereafter. Congratulations! You have much to feel good about and much to look forward to in your future! Just keep applying the skills you've developed here and, soon, these habits for success will become part of who you are, and something you don't even have to think about.

> *Embrace your future!*

We'd also like to plant a seed for a future thought once you've established yourself in your health care career. Remember the help you received from instructors, your network, and maybe a special mentor along the way and consider ways you can give back to the profession and its educational process. Perhaps you'll become a mentor yourself for the next generation of students coming along. While the profession will gain, you'll also feel good about yourself for participating!

## CHAPTER SUMMARY

* Looking at how far you've come can be an encouragement to keep pursuing your dreams.
* It's important to celebrate every accomplishment, no matter how small.
* By thinking about the obstacles you've overcome so far, you can find ways to face future challenges.

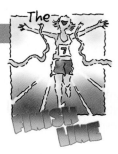

- Evaluate how well you met your goals this semester or term and make plans to avoid problems in the future.
- The knowledge and skills you're learning now will be important in your future career in health care.
- Carefully crafting your résumé and cover letter, and preparing for interviews, helps you land the job you're seeking.

## REVIEW QUESTIONS

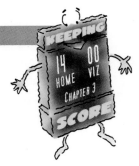

1. Short Essay: Write three to five sentences describing the dreams that brought you to where you are now.
2. What is the biggest obstacle you've overcome so far in your quest for a new career?
3. What goal are you most proud of accomplishing so far?
4. Short Essay: Write three to five sentences about the career knowledge you've gained since beginning school.
5. List skills you have developed in the last 3 years that may be relevant to a future health care career.

## CHAPTER ACTIVITIES

1. Assess Your Success: Make a time line starting from when you first decided you wanted to pursue a health care career and ending with your long-term goal. First, mark the steps you've taken so far, such as narrowing down your career choices, choosing a school, enrolling, registering for courses, adjusting your work schedule, etc. Then, add your intermediate and short-term goals to the timeline. Finally, look at how far you've come and how much farther you need to go.
2. Share the Wealth: Divide into groups of three to five students. Ask each member of the group to talk about the fears he or she had when they first started school and how they found the courage to overcome those fears. Use a chalkboard or poster paper to make a list of fears and how each was overcome so everyone can take notes.
3. Job Search Preparation: Write a résumé based on your work and experience to date, taking note of any areas in which you can become stronger in the period before you actually start making job applications.

# Answers to Keeping Score Questions

## CHAPTER 1
### Review Questions

1. People may choose to continue their education to improve their lifestyles, provide for their families, and gain self-respect.

2. Answers will vary.

3. To be a successful student, look for support from friends and family, coworkers, other students, campus discussion groups, instructors and tutors, academic advisors, and campus resources.

4. A positive attitude is needed to stay motivated to attend classes and study effectively in order to be successful.

5. Answers will vary but should include techniques such as:
   - planning ahead and scheduling your study time
   - reminding yourself of your academic and career goals
   - remembering your successes
   - focusing on the here and now
   - breaking tasks into smaller, manageable pieces
   - avoiding multitasking
   - imitating successful people
   - rewarding yourself for completing significant tasks
   - getting the important things done first
   - networking with other students

6. Goals should be measurable, reachable, and desirable.

7. Answers will vary.

## Chapter Activities

1. Answers will vary but may include:
   - keeping a positive attitude
   - learning to cope with stress

- staying motivated
- setting realistic, manageable goals

2. Answers will vary.

## CHAPTER 2
## Review Questions

1. Answers will vary but may include:
   - You may miss important information for succeeding in the course and for entering your new career.
   - Each time you miss class, you fall further behind.
   - Class time offers information you won't get anywhere else, such as the instructor's own experiences and opinions on what you read in your textbook.
   - You will miss the value of class discussion and interaction with the instructor.
   - Missing classes will affect your grade and make a poor impression on your instructors.
2. It gives you information about grading, homework assignments, course goals, and, sometimes, details about the course schedule.
3. Midterm and final exam dates; due dates for papers and other projects; deadlines for completing each phase of lengthy projects; test dates; your instructors' office hours; important extracurricular and recreational events; deadlines for drop/add; holidays, school vacations, and social commitments.
4. Answers will vary but may include:
   - setting priorities for what's important
   - doing a little bit at a time
   - juggling your deadlines
   - setting realistic goals
   - staying focused
   - being confident about your decisions
   - keeping your goals in mind

## Chapter Activities

1. Answers will vary.

## CHAPTER 3
## Review Questions

1. Answers will vary but may include:
   - setting priorities (and adjust your schedule accordingly)

- simplifying your life (combine errands, avoid TV, use voicemail, learn to say no, etc.)
- learning to relax (massage, yoga, meditation, exercise, relaxation exercises)
- thinking positively (controlling negative thoughts)
- gaining the support of others (family, friends, coworkers, other students, etc.)
- maintaining a healthy body (with regular exercise, a healthful diet, sufficient sleep and rest, and avoiding harmful substances)

2. Healthy foods include:
   - citrus fruits
   - leafy green vegetables
   - whole grains
   - low-fat proteins
   - other foods high in vitamins, potassium, calcium, and magnesium

   Dietary substances to minimize include:
   - sugar
   - salt
   - oils
   - caffeine
   - alcohol

3. Exercise promotes greater health, increases one's energy and mental alertness, helps reduce stress, promotes good sleep, helps with weight management, and improves self-esteem.

4. Answers will vary.

## Chapter Activities

1. Answers will vary.
2. Answers will vary.
3. Answers will vary but may include:
   - using cash instead of a credit card
   - carrying a refillable water bottle instead of buying water
   - bringing along healthy snacks
   - shopping around and compare prices
   - making your own lunches
   - canceling cable TV and watch programs online
   - using free campus and local Wi-Fi spots
   - looking for free fun instead of movies and concerts

## CHAPTER 4
## Review Questions

1. Sitting in front ensures a clear view of the instructor and lets you hear things clearly, as well as encouraging participation and making a good impression.

2. Health professions classrooms tend to get noisy when instructors discuss clinical rotation assignments. If you are unable to hear your instructor over the conversations of other students, you won't know when or where to go for your clinical assignment.

3. Answers will vary but may include that the instructor will notice whether you are paying attention or are engaged in other activities.

4. Learning how to meet and talk to new people now will help you feel more comfortable by the time you have your first real clinical experience.

5. Answers will vary but may include:
   - A study group will help you review and understand course content.
   - Other students may offer tips for how to succeed in a course.
   - You can borrow another student's notes if you must miss a class.
   - Other students provide support by listening to your ideas and sharing their own.

6. Answers will vary; sample answer: Possible challenges include finding trustworthy and helpful people to network with, getting up the nerve to approach them, and then finding a time when everyone is free to get together.

7. Answers will vary but may include differences in race, ethnicity, gender roles, sexual orientation, religion, socioeconomic status, and age.

8. Diversity is an essential part of the rich experience of humanity. Experiencing diversity while in school brings many benefits both in the present and for the future.

## Chapter Activities

1. Answers will vary.
2. Answers will vary.

## CHAPTER 5
## Review Questions

1. By being aware of your learning style, you'll discover ways you can learn more efficiently. This understanding can help you improve your studying and test-taking skills and compensate for your weaknesses.

2. Answers may include: class discussions, class lectures, question-and-answer sessions, giving speeches, reading aloud, study groups, and recorded lectures or speeches.

3. Answers will vary but should be similar to: Thinking critically means analyzing information in order to form judgments about it. The information may be gathered from observations, personal experience, reasoning, or communication.

4. Synthesis and evaluation are higher-level skills that involve judging ideas and information and creatively using information to develop new ideas. Before you can engage these skills, you must first clearly know and comprehend the information—the first two stages of cognitive learning.

## Chapter Activities

1. Answers will vary.

2. Answers will vary.

3. Answers will vary.

## CHAPTER 6
## Review Questions

1. Answers will vary but may include:
   - letting distractions interrupt your train of thought
   - tuning out difficult material
   - allowing your emotions to cloud your thinking
   - assuming the material is boring
   - concentrating on the speaker's quirks
   - letting your mind wander
   - pretending to listen
   - listening only for facts and not ideas
   - trying to write down every word in your notes

2. Answers will vary but may include:
   - summarizing the information in your head
   - memorizing definitions of key terms as your instructor goes over them
   - predicting what information your instructor will cover next

3. A concept map generally works best for note taking with instructors who provide many anecdotes or examples and do not usually follow a strict outline.

4. Review your notes within 24 hours after class to make corrections and add to them while the lecture is still fresh in mind and to help you commit the information to memory.

5. Answers will vary but may include:
   - reading aloud
   - taking notes or drawing graphics as you read
   - writing down any questions you have while reading
   - thinking about how the information you are reading relates to other information you have learned
   - making a note of difficult sections to read a second time

## Chapter Activities

1. Answers will vary.
2. Answers will vary.

## CHAPTER 7
## Review Questions

1. Answers may include:
   - acknowledging your fear and remembering that stage fright is completely normal
   - understanding that the instructor and other students are not looking for faults
   - reassuring yourself that you have something important to say
   - staying focused on *what* you're saying, not *how* others are viewing you
   - practicing repeatedly in advance
   - taking a few deep breaths before beginning
   - speaking loudly and clearly to avoid having to repeat yourself

2. Answers may include: interviews with professors or experts in the field, surveys and statistics, resources on the Internet, unbiased observations, personal experiences (in addition to library research).

3. Using all the steps of the writing (or presentation planning) process helps ensure you succeed in all aspects of the paper or presentation and do not rush through or overlook anything important.

4. Answers may include:
   - scheduling a group meeting as soon as possible to get started
   - brainstorming together about your topic, audience, and goals to ensure everyone is on the same wavelength

- dividing up and assigning specific tasks, such as researching, drafting, developing visual aids, etc.
- choosing a team leader to help keep everyone on schedule, organize meetings, etc.
- while working individually between meetings, everyone should stay in touch
- meeting again before writing the first draft or outlining the presentation, to make final decisions
- working together during the presentation practice or revising of the paper

5. A professional email should be in full sentences with correctly spelled words and reasonable grammar, avoid abbreviations and slang, use a professional name, include a clear subject line, get to the point clearly and concisely, and be neutral in tone.

## Chapter Activities

1. Answers will vary.
2. Answers will vary.

## CHAPTER 8
## Review Questions

1. Get and stay organized by making a place for everything, keeping class materials together in a binder or folder, labeling or color coding materials, organizing class notes, and avoiding the backpack black hole.
2. Answers will vary but may include: practice and repetition, spaced study, making associations, reducing interference, creating lists, or using imagery.
3. They should be Committed Contributors who are Compatible with one another and Considerate of each other.
4. Computerized assessment helps students determine their level of knowledge and focus on what they still need to learn. Assessments help instructors determine their students' progress and adjust the curriculum appropriately if needed.
5. Although a calculator can perform certain mathematical functions, it is only a tool and cannot help you understand what an equation means or how it is used in real life.

## Chapter Activities

1. Answers will vary but may include something similar to:
   - a room where I can shut the door; a large desk so I can spread out my books and notes; a comfortable chair; a window; a CD player so I can listen to soft instrumental music

- move CD player from my bedroom to my study space; clear off the desk so I have room for my study materials; borrow some classical CDs from the local library

2. Tasks could include:

   - Buy supplies (three-ring binders, tabbed dividers or colored card-stock paper, colored marker or pen, three-hole punch, spiral notebooks, etc.).
   - Designate a separate binder for each class.
   - Label tabbed dividers or card stock with appropriate headings (e.g., Schedule, Syllabus, Handouts, Assignments, Notes) and insert one set of dividers in each binder.
   - File all paperwork for each class behind the appropriate tabs.
   - Insert a supply of blank notebook paper behind the "Notes" tab in each binder (or use a separate spiral-bound notebook to take notes for each class).
   - Clean out your backpack after the first day of class. File any stray papers in their appropriate binders.

3. Answers will vary.

## CHAPTER 9
## Grade Calculation Practice

1. 90.9%
2. 82.5%
3. 85%
4. 92.6%
5. 92%

## Review Questions

1. Answers will vary but may include: Preparation is most important—study thoroughly, know what to study. Keep to your normal schedule and don't cut out eating right or exercising. Budget your time well during the test and try to answer every question, even if only in outline form.

2. Talk to the instructor and look at old versions of the test.

3. When you're writing your outline, start with your thesis statement. Use a five-paragraph format to organize the body of your outline, including the introduction, your main points and supporting details, and your conclusion. It's important to write an outline because content and organization typically count for most of your test grade. If you run out of time and can't finish your essay, you can at least show your outline

to let your instructor know that time was the problem, not comprehension.

4. Answers will vary but may include:

- Words and phrases like *except, not,* and *all of the following* provide important clues.
- Try to answer the question before looking at the answer choices and then match your answer to the best of the choices.
- Use a process of elimination to narrow your answer choices, first crossing out ones that are clearly incorrect.
- Be alert for "attractive distracters" that look like the correct answer but aren't.
- Work quickly—don't use too much time checking and double-checking questions you think you answered correctly.

## Chapter Activities

1. List could include actions such as: I want to start riding my bike again and I want to try tai chi. For the bike, I'll need to get that front tire changed and buy a bike helmet. For tai chi, I could buy a video that shows me the basics, then practice it in the backyard.

2. Answers will vary.

3. Answers will vary.

## CHAPTER 10
## Review Questions

1. Answers will vary.

2. Answers will vary but should include specifics on your chosen career from one of the websites listed in the chapter.

3. Answers will vary.

4. Important personal characteristics include: caring, integrity, dependability, trustworthiness, teamwork, openness to change, flexibility and willingness to keep learning, and good personal health.

5. Characteristics of a profession include: specialized education and the competence of practitioners, being self-regulating, active membership in a professional association, and networking among professionals.

## Chapter Activities

1. Answers will vary.

2. Answers will vary.

3. Answers will vary.

## CHAPTER 11
## Review Questions

1. Use your school's skills lab.

2. If you try to do something you're not qualified to do, you could make a mistake and possibly harm a patient or get into legal trouble. But if you always work within your limits, you'll be protecting yourself, the patients, and the facility where you work.

3. Your mentor is someone who can be a role model, share their own experiences, answer your questions, and provide a private audience for your concerns.

4. To prepare for beginning the clinical experience:
   - Know the dress code.
   - Know the equipment.
   - Know your mentor.
   - Know the clinic.

5. Answers will vary; sample answer: Health care is all about teamwork and it's important to show you can work successfully with others. The work of every member of the team is important to other members of the team providing patient care.

## Chapter Activities

1. Answers may vary but can include questions such as:
   - Where do I buy my uniform?
   - What happens if I accidentally break a HIPAA rule?
   - What if I make mistakes during a procedure?

2. Answers will vary.

## CHAPTER 12
## Review Questions and Chapter Activities

Answers will vary.

# Index